Negligent by Design

NEGLIGENT BY DESIGN

ANTI-BLACKNESS IN AMERICAN MEDICINE AND HOW TO ADDRESS IT

VANESSA GRUBBS, MD

North Atlantic Books
Huichin, unceded Ohlone land
aka Berkeley, California

North Atlantic Books
Huichin, unceded Ohlone land
2526 Martin Luther King Jr Way
Berkeley, CA 94704 USA
www.northatlanticbooks.com

Cover art © Caelestiss, ulimi, and kyoshino via Getty Images
Cover design by Jess Morphew
Book design by Happenstance Type-O-Rama

Printed in the United States of America

Negligent by Design: Anti-Blackness in American Medicine and How to Address It is sponsored and published by North Atlantic Books, an educational nonprofit that collaborates with partners to develop cross-cultural perspectives; nurture holistic views of art, science, the humanities, and healing; and seed personal and global transformation by publishing work on the relationship of body, spirit, and nature.

North Atlantic Books' publications are distributed to the US trade and internationally by Penguin Random House Publishers Services. For further information, visit our website at www.northatlanticbooks.com.

The authorized representative in the EU for product safety and compliance is Eucomply OÜ, Pärnu mnt 139b-14, 11317 Tallinn, Estonia, hello@eucompliancepartner.com, +33757690241.

Library of Congress Cataloging-in-Publication Data

Names: Grubbs, Vanessa author
Title: Negligent by design : anti-blackness in American medicine and how to address it / Vanessa Grubbs, MD.
Description: Berkeley, California : North Atlantic Books, [2025] | Includes bibliographical references and index.
Identifiers: LCCN 2025412027 (print) | LCCN 2025002466 (ebook) | ISBN 9798889842354 trade paperback | ISBN 9798889842361 ebook
Subjects: LCSH: Discrimination in medical care--United States | African Americans--Medical care | African Americans--Health and hygiene | Health and race--United States | Medical personnel--Malpractice--United States
Classification: LCC RA448.5.B53 G78 2025 (print) | LCC RA448.5.B53 (ebook) | DDC 362.1089/96073--dc23/eng/20250609
LC record available at https://lccn.loc.gov/2025412027
LC ebook record available at https://lccn.loc.gov/2025002466

1 2 3 4 5 6 7 8 9 KPC 30 29 28 27 26 25

For all the little Black ones
who dream of being a doctor.

You belong.

CONTENTS

ACKNOWLEDGMENTS

I will forever be thankful to the people who trusted me with their stories about Medicine. They were all so poignant, whether they be from patient, student, or physician perspectives.

When I met my literary agent, Kate Johnson, in 2018, I had a quirky fiction idea that she fully supported. And when that project was pushed to the back burner for this one a year later, she was still on board. I am immensely grateful for her steadfast encouragement.

Thank you, Shawn Ginwright, for e-introducing me to Tim McKee of North Atlantic Books, who found my proposal for this book intriguing after pretty much everybody else decided to pass. A special thanks to my editor Jas Respess, who was so very patient with me but delivered the tough love I needed to get this book done.

A special shout-out to Stacey Senat, Black Doc Village's program manager and first employee. She helped keep me organized and sane through our first major research project. She is the best hype woman a girl could ever ask for, with frequent reminders that I am "that B."

Finally, I thank my husband, love of my life, and best friend, Robert Phillips, for being the chill to my no chill. Don't forget to remind me that I said writing this book felt like giving birth after five years of labor without an epidural should I ever hint at wanting to write another one.

NEGLIGENT MEDICINE

Stranded

Little black one
What you doing here?
Did you lose your way
Or did you think you were
Finding a way?
Ain't nobody like you been
In these here parts
As far as the mind can see
Cain't you tell by the way we smile
There's no need to worry
We've done this before
Little black one

> —*Vanessa Grubbs*
> *Duke University School of Medicine*
> *1994*

At the beginning of my nephrology faculty tenure at the University of California, San Francisco (UCSF), I was one of the "good ones." I knew my place—sitting at a bench in the back of an abandoned lab, grateful that a man with "Dirty White Boy" tattooed across his torso gave me legitimacy. I was so good that I abandoned the research topic that brought me to nephrology for work that offended no one. Nobody took issue with me trying to show severe gum disease was a risk factor for worsening kidney disease. But when I proposed to uncover and fix the reasons why Black people were half as likely to get a kidney transplant as White people, my mentor refused to sponsor me. When we spoke, my boss forgot he had assigned me an office too narrow for a meeting. I'm not sure if it was winning the research grants, the book deal, or the belief that people in high places had my back, but within a few years, I forgot my small place so much so that those in power used a tweet to try to put me back in it.

I was away at some work conference, communicating by email with a trainee about one of my home dialysis patients who had developed a dialysis-related infection. Two weeks prior, this same trainee had given me the *oh how cute you think you have something to teach me* eyes in clinic, so I wasn't entirely surprised when he chose to bypass my instructions for the patient's care and follow those from the senior male attending physician overseeing the inpatient consult service. This attending physician hadn't cared for home dialysis patients in 15 years.

Being treated with this type of disregard was nothing new to me. Nor to other minoritized women faculty. In division meetings, we all had voiced how trainees often automatically regarded White/White-adjacent male physicians with a level of respect they rarely afforded minoritized female physicians. The White and non-Black male physicians shrugged us off because they "didn't see it." So, with two incidents in short order and our attempts to be heard within the institution being ignored, I had enough and wanted to initiate a broader conversation.

In a short Twitter thread, I sarcastically asked why a nephrology fellow would choose to take the recommendation of another attending about the treatment plan for *my* patient after I instructed them on what to do. Not wanting to fully out the individuals involved, I ended with my usual Twitter snark: "Happy to provide demographics if that helps."

Unfortunately, it was as if I had just shouted into the wind. After a few hours, my tweets only had one "like." And since I wanted to avoid the usual Twitter off-topic devolvement into a clinical debate rather than focusing on the real issue, I deleted them.

When I returned, the trainee had rotated to another hospital, and the patient was being treated. I moved on.

Turns out I didn't delete the tweets fast enough. And I was the only one who moved on. Two months later, I learned someone had seen the tweets and deciphered the identities of unnamed individuals I referred to. It escalated from there. But I was not made aware there was a problem until *after* all the fellows, the fellowship director, the division of nephrology chiefs from our three affiliated hospital sites, the department of medicine chiefs at my hospital and the university hospital, the head of the university's Academic Affairs office, and the unnamed individuals had all discussed the matter. Only then was I asked for my perspective. *Two months later.*

"So, tell me about the fight with the fellow," said Neil Powe, chief of medicine at San Francisco General Hospital, where my clinical work and research program were based.

I was taken aback, my brows furrowed in confusion. "What fight?"

The meeting was held around a small round table in Neil's office. Neil and I sat across from each other, and he gestured to my direct supervisor, David, the chief of nephrology at San Francisco General, who was seated between us.

I looked at David with both *what fight* and *what the fuck* eyes since a fight had not come up in our meeting the day before, when I handed him my resignation letter. At that time, I had intended to transfer to the Division of Palliative Care, where my research mentor and more like-minded colleagues resided.

I realized I was in serious trouble over a tweet and became increasingly angry because, in those last two months, I had attended meetings and clinics and interacted with people as my work routine entailed, completely oblivious to the fact that I was the subject of detailed conversations in my hospital, division, and the far corners of university leadership. I was humiliated.

"You misconstrued the incident," my superiors reprimanded. Because the others involved weren't White, they denied any bias was at play. They said this as if anti-Blackness isn't global. As if anti-Blackness can't be communicated through body language and actions.

I was ostracized. Fellows would no longer have to work under my supervision because they feared I might take to Twitter about "imagined racism." Funny enough, that decision was reversed a week later—perhaps because I told them I didn't see that as punishment. I preferred to see my patients independently, and I found no joy in trying to teach people who assumed I had no knowledge to share. More likely, I suspect the decision was reversed because they had something else in mind. With an HR representative in the room, I was asked to sign a disclosure that I would never tweet about trainees again.

By then, I was done. They had taken away my dream of becoming a full professor—the peak of academia. I would not allow them to take my voice too.

My dream formed in 2012 when I sat in the middle of a nearly full auditorium listening to the UCSF Department of Medicine chair's State of the Department of Medicine lecture. He showed the obligatory diversity slide of all faculty by race and academic title on the large screen. Sadly, but not surprisingly, I watched him point out the handful of black dots representing Black academics who had made it to full professorship. I envisioned myself becoming one of those black dots. That would have made me the first Black professor in my nephrology division's 50-year existence.

Instead, I decided to leave UCSF shortly after my promotion to associate professor in September 2019, four years shy of the full professor goal. I decided to leave not because, as many might assume, I couldn't do it like some failed affirmative action experiment, proving that I was there primarily because, as a Black female, I had been graded on a diversity curve and my merits were not enough. An assumption my high school science teacher first introduced me to as the reason why I could get into a school like Duke University. An assumption that visited often and kept me company between every standardized exam.

It had become apparent that even though I had been awarded two competitive leadership fellowships, my home institution did not see me that way. My efforts to lead felt dismissed, undermined, and usurped. I felt that had someone non-Black come along and said the same words and performed the same efforts to improve patient care, the response would have been much different. Similarly, I believe the reaction would have been different had I tweeted about something other than implicit bias. If I had been a senior White male physician who berated staff and trainees to the point of tears for what he perceived as stupidity for years, instead of a Black woman tweeting about racism, I would have been named division chief.

After some reflection, I admit I should not have been tweeting the day the situation happened. Though I mentioned no names and intended to discuss a general issue rather than target a specific person, it was shortsighted not to foresee that others in the small program would see it and be able to identify the people involved. I should have waited longer to vent. I should have further de-identified the tweet. I should have known people were trolling my social media. I should have known my actions would spark outrage and retaliation, instead of open and honest conversation.

However, I also assert that the appropriate reaction to my wrongdoing would have been for a supervisor to talk to me about the situation when they became aware of it and instruct me not to tweet identifiably again. Instead, one short Twitter thread in my 10 years as nephrology faculty, and 6 years after joining Twitter, was met with my boss reporting it to his boss who escalated it to the highest echelons of the institution. They whispered behind my back for two months before informing me of their plan to invalidate, ostracize, and silence me, and all before asking me anything.

I was reminded of stories of Black girls around the country whose slights were met with excessive reactions. Stories like that of Grace, the 15-year-old

Black girl in Michigan who was jailed for two months because she didn't turn in her online homework. Like 6-year-old Kaia Rolle in Florida, who was hand-cuffed for throwing a tantrum, and an 11-year-old Black girl in New Mexico who a police officer shoved against a wall and slammed to the ground because she took too many milks in the school cafeteria and picked at a sign taped to a door.

On a less overt scale, the response to my wrongdoing was similarly excessive and emblematic of society's way of overreacting to the actions of Black girls and women—especially because I suggest bias/racism was at hand. To imply some-one's actions were racist, subconscious though they may be, is immediately met with defensiveness and vehement denial, with no space or desire left over to discuss the actions at hand. But I won't hold my breath waiting for any of those involved in the overreaction to admit they were wrong.

"I just wish you had come talk to me first," David offered as an alternative to my tweeting.

"Me too, David. I wish you had come talk to me first too," I said solemnly.

No, I was not interested in staying somewhere I couldn't be heard, let alone appreciated or supported. The handling of this situation unveiled to me an institutional mindset that said, "You forgot your place, little Black one." That message made me no longer want to be part of an institution that could only hear me if I was praising it or otherwise making it look good. I wanted noth-ing to do with an institution that would treat me incommensurately with my wrongdoing yet look away from, and outright deny, actions perpetrated against me. In their eyes, I had repeatedly committed the unforgivable offense of implying someone's actions were racist, subconscious though they may be. And this latest one was in the public eye. It should not have surprised me that I was met with defensiveness, denial, and retribution.

My decision to leave was a conscious choice, but in truth, I felt pushed out as much as I felt pulled to pursue other interests—like writing this book. So when a prospective editor read an early proposal for this book project and was disappointed in how I framed the topic, they asked why I didn't go straight at the issue.

"Just say Medicine is racist," they said.

"Because I'm a Black woman," I answered. "I don't get to say or write such things. Not and be heard."

So to move the conversation forward before folks immediately knee-jerk into self-defense cries about how they *don't have a racist bone in their body* and how *there is a Black person in their family*, I've decided to frame this subject matter in a way more people may be able to hear it:

American Medicine is negligent. By design. Yes, the whole damn institution. At least when it comes to race, particularly Black race.

In my first book, *Hundreds of Interlaced Fingers*, I touched on how race factored into medicine and how every case presentation was expected to start with the patient's age, race, and gender.[1] I explained how Black race has been used in the estimation of kidney function and how there were no Black nephrology faculty available to me at UCSF when I was seeking a research mentor at the start of my fellowship.

At the time, I didn't want to be viewed as just another Black doctor hyper-focused on "disparities" and I was still under the notion that palliative care, my non-offensive research focus, was the great equalizer when it came to race. Because everybody dies, it doesn't matter if you're Black, White, Yellow, Red, or Purple, I wrote. Well, bless my naïve heart, because while it's true everybody dies, I've come to realize that in America, race matters in everything because race is, quite literally, what this country was built on through chattel slavery.

Due to that realization, this book became a wide look and a deep dive into race in American Medicine. There will be no touching, tiptoeing, or lightly grazing on racial negligence in these pages.

The *Merriam-Webster* dictionary defines being *negligent* as "failing to exercise the care that a reasonably prudent person would exercise in similar circumstances."[2]

This is not to be confused with *medical negligence,* a legal term meaning a medical professional's action (or failure to act) that deviates from the accepted medical standard of care. The *standard of care* for Black people in this country has always been and continues to be negligent, by design.

This book describes how Medicine is negligent in three distinct ways: race based, race disregarded, and race denied. While these may seem conflicting, they are united in creating worse health outcomes for Black people.

In the first part, "Race Based," I describe the history behind race science and how it touches every medical specialty. I delve into the evidence underlying "correcting" for Black race in estimating kidney function and how staunchly continuing to do so was defended.

In the second part, "Race Disregarded," I explore how Medicine ignores the aspects of race that do matter. From diagnosing rashes on darker skin tones, to listening to lived experiences, to acknowledging why diversity matters.

In the third part, "Race Denied," I discuss the ways Medicine copes with its feelings of distress, anxiety, and sadness when confronted with the realities of racism. I describe Medicine's defensive behaviors, from the *denial* that they could be racist and the *distraction* of White tears and insistence that *all* diversity matters, not just racial diversity, to the actual *destruction* of individual careers that dare threaten their image of themselves.

In the fourth and final part, "From Negligent to Conscientious," I describe how Medicine's current actions to address its negligent treatment of Black people amount to little more than a *placebo*—a harmless prescription in the form of procedures such as forming diversity committees and releasing statements condemning police violence that primarily, if not solely, serve Medicine's own psychological benefit. Then I describe what Medicine could and should do to stop its negligence (if it was really about that life): commit to *cultural humility,* as defined in the original 1998 article, coauthored by Drs. Melanie Tervalon and Jann Murray-García, and published in the *Journal of Health Care for the Poor and Underserved*—an approach that describes a pathway to equity and inclusion. A "whatever it takes" approach for Medicine to uproot the feelings of fear, inadequacy, and insecurity that led to its negligent behavior, because only in doing so would it be able to recruit and retain the diverse physician workforce necessary to get better health outcomes for marginalized communities.

But don't get it twisted; my reframing of Medicine as negligent is by no means a way to make it palatable for the willfully ignorant. No, this book is not another feel-good, kumbaya, Rodney King–esque "can't we just all get along" plea. It is an undeniable truth-telling. *Negligent by Design* is a call to action that concludes with a playbook on how we can force Medicine to behave differently—regardless of what the powers that be say.

This book will strengthen advocates' resolve, inform all people of what is happening throughout the halls of Medicine, and show them what they can do about it. A growing number of us have already started. This book will invite and instruct the convinced reader to pick up a hammer, since, as Audre Lorde reminds us, "The master's tools will never dismantle the master's house."[3]

PART I
RACE BASED

CHAPTER 1

RACE SCIENCE

In 2013, when Castle Redmond's girlfriend told him about his loud snoring and periods of not breathing altogether, he sought help. A home-based sleep study had diagnosed him with sleep apnea. If left untreated, sleep apnea can lead to abnormal heart rhythms, heart failure, worsening memory, erectile dysfunction, pulmonary hypertension, and even death. The conventional treatment is continuous positive airway pressure (CPAP), a steady stream of air pushed at a prescribed force from a machine resembling an old-school radio. The CPAP machine takes up most of the space on a typical nightstand. It pushes air into a hose connected to a mask that covers the person's mouth and nose and is strapped around their head. But after trying nearly a dozen different CPAP masks without success, Castle sought an alternative. "I'm a restless sleeper," he recalled. "None of them would stay on through the night."

Somewhere along the way, he had read about a mouthguard treatment. He had self-diagnosed that the problem was his jaw falling back during the night and causing airway obstruction, but he sought the opinion of a pulmonologist at an academic medical center, hoping to be treated with state-of-the-art technology. He was pleased that they first scheduled him for a sleep study in a real sleep center instead of relying on the janky DIY home study. A few months after the repeat study confirmed his diagnosis of severe sleep apnea, Castle returned to the clinic to discuss the next steps with the pulmonologist. At this appointment, he shared his desire to try a mouthguard.

Castle described the pulmonologist who entered the room as the kind of doctor you might see on TV: a White man who looked to be in his sixties, of average height, a bit overweight, and with only remnants of salt-and-pepper hair on his balding head. He shook Dr. Made-For-TV's hand, taking in the contrast between the doctor and himself before taking a seat. Castle stood six-foot-four and had weighed about 250 pounds since his college linebacker days. With his shaven head and skin the color of deep caramel, he presented as a Black man unambiguously. It did not often occur to strangers that he was biracial.

Though they met in a clinic exam room, Castle wasn't examined.

"It won't work for you," Dr. Made-For-TV offered when Castle said he wanted to try a mouthguard. "Black people's jaws protrude forward," the doctor added. "You know, like Patrick Ewing, as a reference point for you."

With sincerity in his eyes, Dr. Made-For-TV motioned his right hand back and forth at his own jaw to demonstrate exactly what he meant, as if Castle, a man with a law degree, might not know the definition of the word *protrude*.

It is true that mouthguards, or oral appliances, are designed to either pull the lower jaw forward or hold the tongue forward so it doesn't fall back and block the airway. The lower jaw, the mandible, is the strongest bone in the human face and holds the lower teeth in place. Excluding the three tiny bones in the inner ear that move when sound waves vibrate the eardrum, the lower jaw is the only bone in the skull that can move. The hinge joints that connect it to the temporal bones, which protect the middle and inner ears, allow the mouth to open and close, move from side to side, and forward and back. So it makes sense that if a person's lower jaw can't move forward at least six millimeters, or about a quarter inch, a mouthguard designed to pull the lower jaw forward will not work.

It is also true that Patrick Ewing, one of the best NBA players of all time, has a protruding lower jaw. With his seven-foot frame and wide upturned nose, Ewing was often ridiculed and compared to an ape by opposing teams' fans during his four years playing for Georgetown University—a comparison emanating from a Medicine-fortified legacy of associating Black people with primates. Journalist Gary Pomerantz reported in a 1983 *Washington Post* article how Villanova fans raised a bedsheet that read "Ewing Is An Ape" and, when Ewing ran out for pregame introductions, someone from the crowd flung a banana peel onto the court. Blatant racism aside, it makes sense that an apparatus designed to pull the lower jaw forward would not work for Patrick Ewing or anyone with a jaw like Patrick Ewing's.

What is not true is that all Black people have an underbite.

Medicine would argue that one physician's ignorance says nothing about Medicine on the whole, because that is what Medicine does—takes credit for every example of its brilliance but distances itself from any semblance of shortcomings. Some would say how ridiculous it is that a pulmonologist could believe that *all* Black people had such a protruding lower jaw that direct examination of the patient in front of them is unnecessary and mouthguards were never even worth trying. But Medicine trained him. Medicine established the foundation by doing the work that started the comparison of Black people to apes. That "science" lent a legitimacy that permeated Medicine and the greater society.

This idea can be traced back to the writings of Samuel Morton, an American physician who was held in high esteem as both a physician and a scientist for his work dubbed "craniometry" on more than 900 human skulls. These skulls were collected from various "suppliers"—a sordid history all on its own. His work was so highly regarded that upon his death in 1851, the *Charleston Medical Journal* heralded him as the South's "benefactor for aiding most materially in giving to the negro his true position as an inferior race."[1]

In Josiah Clark Nott's *Types of Mankind*, published in 1854, Morton is quoted: "Although Negro races present considerable variety in their cranial conformations, yet they all possess certain unmistakeable [*sic*] traits in common, marking them as Negroes, and distinguishing them from all other species of man. Prognathous [protruding] jaws, narrow elongated forms, receding forehead, large posterior development, small internal capacity, characterize the whole group craniologically." To solidify the agenda of not merely describing, but ascribing hierarchical meaning, Morton continues: "If we take the profile view of the European face . . . we shall find that it can be divided by horizontal lines into four equal parts. . . . It is especially in this deviation from the normal measurement that the human features become coarse and ugly. In a comparison of the Negro head with this ideal, we get the surprising result that the rule . . . is a regular increase in length from above downwards. . . . All zoologists are aware of the great difference in the formation of the heads of . . . orang-outans [*sic*] . . . particularly the jaw."[2]

Although Morton was later renamed as the "father of scientific racism," his sentiments continued in the literature, most recently in nurse and anthropologist Theresa Overfield's critically acclaimed textbook *Biological Variation in Health and Illness: Race, Age, and Sex Differences* (2nd Edition), which was published in 1995. In it, Overfield writes assertively: "Because teeth may indicate developmental, hygienic, and nutritional adequacy, health workers should note the differences that occur by race. . . . Differences in tooth size among races help explain the differential occurrence of prognathism. Tooth size, dental arch, and jaw size are positively correlated; hence prognathism is seen more frequently in Blacks and Orientals."[3]

Overfield arrived at this conclusion by comparing tooth measurements from two studies: one from Kubota and colleagues on Nigerian and Japanese children and adults published in 1993, and one from Anderson and colleagues on White Canadian teenagers published in 1977. So on the basis of a few hundred people in Nigeria and Japan, generalizations are applied to all Black and Asian people. While these may seem like dusty, obsolete texts, they serve as the foundation that has informed, and continues to live in, today's clinical world.

Castle blinked hard and furrowed his brow as he tried to process the doctor's words. He was used to people making assumptions about his Blackness in the world, but he was dismayed to see he needed to be conscious of race in a doctor's office too. He immediately lost all faith in this doctor's ability to help him. He felt his very well-being was in the control of a physician—perhaps an entire health care system—who was incapable of seeing beyond his race-based assumptions.

"Yeah, well, my mom is White," Castle finally said, playing into the doctor's assumption to prove him wrong.

"Oh," said Dr. Made-For-TV, wrinkling his forehead in surprise. "Well, maybe it'll work then," he added.

This response further underscores that the legacy of the "father of scientific racism" lives on in modern-day physicians like Dr. Made-For-TV and through researchers who continuously look for and report differences based on small populations of Black and White people. From this legacy of debunked "science," they take away a message that Black people are completely different and separate from White people and that all Black people are, more or less, the same.

In Castle's case, Dr. Made-For-TV questioned his entire analysis upon learning that Castle's mother was White. Yet all that Dr. Made-For-TV documented in his clinical note of his encounter with Castle was that he had "discussed in detail that it might not be of benefit to him in view of retrognathia [i.e., overbite] and severe sleep apnea," though he had never examined the position of Castle's lower jaw.

The encounter engendered a mistrust that prevented Castle from seeking the help of another pulmonologist for several years. This time, the pulmonologist who entered the room was a White woman who appeared to be in her sixties as well. She examined Castle and gave an opinion that validated what he believed to be the problem all along—that his lower jaw sliding back during his sleep was causing the airway obstruction. He shared with her what Dr. Made-For-TV said.

"Hmph. That's weird," she responded. Castle studied her face, but he couldn't tell if she was silently condemning or reconciling it. But he was glad that she at least examined his actual jaw and was prescribing a mouthguard. He just hoped her prescription was in time to prevent the harms of untreated sleep apnea in the years' delay in care.

Castle's story is just one example of Medicine's negligence toward Black people. It should come as no surprise that Medicine believes in White supremacy—that Whiteness is biologically superior and should, therefore, reign over all others. Medicine has been at the forefront in the effort to "prove" that the races are distinct, and the White race is better, and not just some shit colonizers made up to justify their raping and pillaging.

Within Medicine, it was German physician Johann Blumenbach during the Enlightenment era of the 17th and 18th centuries who followed the work of Carolus Linnaeus, a Swedish botanist, to taxonomize humans into biologically distinct races by consolidating their observations with travelogues of European colonizers. Their proposals for biologically distinctive human varieties, or hierarchized "races," became entrenched as knowledge and served to legitimize colonization.

This is how the various skull measurements led to pronouncements about intelligence. Medicine's actions to "prove" White supremacy were in keeping with sentiments from the soon-to-be third US president, Thomas Jefferson. In his *Notes on the State of Virginia*, first published in 1784, Jefferson made physical and genetic observations of Black people, asserting that Black and White bodies functioned differently. People of African descent, he said, "have less hair on the face and body. They secrete less by the [kidneys], and more by the glands of the skin." Additionally, Black people were "more tolerant of heat, and less so of cold, than the whites." He claimed Black people also had a different "structure in the pulmonary apparatus," but were also "as brave, and more adventuresome" as White people. He attributed this excess risky behavior to "a want of fore-thought [*sic*], which prevents their seeing a danger till it be present," essentially arguing Black people processed information more slowly than White people. To a certain extent, he believed Black people's "faculties of memory, reason, and imagination" were somewhat commensurate to White people's, but he saw Black people as "much inferior," and "in imagination they are dull, tasteless, and anomalous."[4]

In Medicine, Jefferson's most direct influence can be seen in the writings of Samuel Cartwright, a slaveowner and respected physician in his time. He took the baton and sprinted with it in his 1851 publication, *Report on the Diseases and Physical Peculiarities of the Negro Race*. In it, he describes a disease he called "drapetomania," which tied into the long history of Black people in Africa before enslavement, to justify slavery by claiming Black people had no contributions to world "civilization." In his estimation, Black people "prefer the same kind of government, which we call slavery, but which is actually an improvement on the government of their forefathers, as it gives them more tranquility and sensual enjoyment, expands the mind and improves the morals." Without Western "civilization," he says, Black people would "relapse into barbarism."[5]

It was the assumption that Black people are inherently different in health and disease—and specifically the belief that Black people had inferior intelligence—that gave us the US Public Health Service's Tuskegee Study of Untreated Syphilis in the Negro Male. Better known as "Tuskegee," because USPHS is a mouthful and America attempted to suggest it was a study located in a single historically Black college and time, rather than the government-sanctioned decades-long experiment it was.

According to Harriet Washington's *Medical Apartheid: The Dark History of Medical Experimentation on Black Americans from Colonial Times to the Present*, Medicine believed that the devastating neurologic effects of late-stage syphilis (a sexually transmitted infection) in White people would be largely absent in the "less evolved nervous systems" of Black people.[6] So it was this lie that justified observing some 600 poor Black men, their wives, and children—including the 399 who had syphilis—for nearly three decades *after* penicillin was widely available. All while telling the participants they were being treated for "bad blood."

The study began in 1932. By 1972, 28 participants had died of syphilis and 100 more from syphilis-related complications. As a result of the whistleblowing of Peter Buxtun, the Public Health Service formed a committee in the mid-1960s to respond to his concerns that the study was unethical. The committee decided to continue tracking the participants until all of them were dead, the autopsies performed, and the data analyzed. It was sometime after 2004 when the final study participant died. Nevertheless, it took a quarter century since the committee's formation for the government to issue a formal apology, delivered by President Bill Clinton in 1997.

The general public only became aware of Medicine's belief in the inferior intelligence in Black people when *The New York Times* published journalist Ken Belson's story "Black Former NFL Players Say Racial Bias Skews Concussion Payouts" in August 2020. Although chronic traumatic encephalopathy (CTE)—a progressive and fatal brain disease linked to repeated blows to the head, only diagnosable by brain autopsy after death—was first described in 1928 among boxers and more recently among football players by Dr. Bennet Omalu in 2002, it probably wasn't known to most people until Will Smith uttered the meme-worthy words "Tell the truth!" to a National Football League (NFL) official in his depiction of Omalu's discovery in the 2015 movie *Concussion.*

In his article, Belson recounts retired NFL player Najeh Davenport's story. Davenport played in the NFL from 2002 to 2008. After a neurological exam in 2019 confirmed the reduction of his "use of language and executive functioning—or ability to manage and regulate his mental processes," he applied for and was awarded compensation from the NFL. But then the league appealed the award, claiming that when Davenport's scores were recalculated accounting for his race—something the league called an "industry standard"—Davenport was not impaired in any category, and ineligible for a payout. Said another way, because retired Black NFL players were presumed to be inherently dumber than retired White NFL players, when a White player was considered impaired enough for compensation, a Black player at the same level of impairment would not be "sick enough."[7]

This "industry standard" is based upon the Heaton norms, named after Robert K. Heaton, a neuropsychologist at UC San Diego. In developing these norms, researchers found that race/ethnicity in neuropsychological impairment was unrelated to other characteristics, specifically age, education, and gender, in Black and White participants. They believed "normative sampling and standards may lead to neuropsychological misclassification and may particularly contribute to misdiagnosis of African Americans"[8]—that is, saying they were impaired when they weren't.

The researchers acknowledge that "score differences between African American and Caucasian groups may include academic exposure, education quality, academic resources, acculturation, socioeconomic status, social exposure, 'test wiseness,' societal discrimination . . . and lifelong experiences contributing to low group and self-expectations." Rather than delving deeper into these areas of research, however, the Heaton norms researchers decided that assuming all Black people were similar enough across these factors to simply "correct" for race was good enough.

As Maya Angelou said, "When you know better, do better," so one would think that players just starting out would be tested over time to allow comparison with themselves, rather than with an arbitrary definition of "normal." Then again, maybe neither Medicine nor the NFL wants to know the truth.

Early beliefs also held that Black people did not feel pain or anxiety—a notion that helped justify the treatment of the enslaved. At that time, medical practitioners conducting surgical procedures did not feel the need to worry about providing anesthesia to someone who feels no pain. What concerned them was knowing if the differences between Black and White skin was limited to melanin. In the autobiographical account *Slave Life in Georgia: A Narrative of the Life, Sufferings, and Escape of John Brown* published in 1855, Brown described how blisters were applied to his hands, legs, and feet every two weeks for nine months to "ascertain how deep [his] black skin went."[9]

In *Medical Apartheid*, Harriet Washington details statements from physicians like Charles White who declared, "Negroes bear surgical operations much better than White people and what would be the cause of insupportable pain for White men, a Negro would almost disregard . . . [I have] amputated the legs of many Negroes, who have held the upper part of the limb themselves."[10] Dr. James Johnson, editor of the London *Medico-Chirurgical Review*, said of Kentucky surgeon Ephraim McDowell's writings about his surgeries, "When we come to reflect that all the women operated upon in Kentucky, except one, were Negresses and that these people will bear anything with nearly if not quite as much impunity as dogs and rabbits, our wonder is lessened."[11]

Perhaps the most sinister yet contradictory accounts were from Dr. James Marion Sims of Alabama. His efforts to perfect vesicovaginal fistula—abnormal holes between the vagina and colon or bladder caused by prolonged childbirth through a small pelvis, which leaves the individual with the shame and odor of constantly leaking stool or urine—earned him the moniker "the father of modern gynecology." But that he did so by experimenting on enslaved Black women without anesthesia in the 1840s rightfully earns him the title of sadist in my humble opinion. He argued that the Black women felt no pain, but the young White doctors who initially assisted Sims by holding down the enslaved women soon abandoned him, no longer able to bear the blood-curdling screams induced by his incisions.

While the reasonable person would expect those more prone to developing these fistulas are the barely pubescent girls raped by their enslavers or through forced marriage, Medicine ultimately found a way to blame race for obstetric complications. A choice that ultimately affected patient care.

As Vyas and her colleagues detail in their 2019 commentary "Challenging the Use of Race in the Vaginal Birth After Cesarean Section Calculator," the classification of pelvis types by race traces back to the late 1800s.[12] The most influential description of pelvic types stems from Caldwell and Moloy's classification proposed in 1933, which reduced vast anatomic variation to four subtypes: gynecoid, anthropoid, android, and platypelloid. Caldwell and Moloy cited the 1886 published work of Turner, the first to describe the anthropoid pelvis as a "degraded or animalized arrangement seen in the lower races." All of this work lives on in modern-day textbooks like *Williams Obstetrics*, currently on its 26th edition, published in 2022.

It also lent legitimacy to the use of race in developing the Vaginal Birth After Cesarean (VBAC) calculator, which until 2021 was used to decide who should be allowed to try giving birth vaginally lest they rupture their uterus. The VBAC was developed from the outcomes of roughly 7,600 pregnant women with prior C-sections participating in the study between 1999 and 2002. Race was the only nonmeasurable variable that made it into the final algorithm. As opposed to the social advantages of Whiteness in America, according to the researchers, simply being Black or Hispanic negatively affects the probability of success nearly as much as the positive affect of having a past vaginal birth. As a result, clinicians are less likely to allow a Black or Hispanic person to *try* giving birth naturally—even though natural birth avoids surgical complications and allows faster recovery time.

A young Black ob-gyn I spoke with shared her perspective on the topic. Despite her understanding of the calculator's racist roots, as a resident physician, she felt obligated to report the calculation when presenting patients to her supervisors. Doing so demonstrated her knowledge of the latest tools for best clinical practices. But what the practice demonstrated to her was that birthing centers could do several C-sections in the time it took to have one person laboring for hours and hours. In this way, the low reimbursement rates of Medi-Cal could still generate reasonable income *and* be justified by "science." The fact that Black birthing people had nearly four times the mortality of their White counterparts regardless of patient income, insurance, education, comorbid conditions, or prenatal care is seemingly dismissed as just another hazard of ape-like pelvises.[13]

I might have been one of those Black women affected by this calculator. In 1999 I was looking forward to feeling my cervix open and bravely bearing down to push my son into the world. I let go of the first part of my dream when, after four hours of getting a firsthand lesson in what "blinding pain" meant as every contraction brought a bright white flash that eclipsed my view of the room, my cervix had only dilated from 3 to 4 centimeters. Knowing that 10 centimeters was the goal, I politely asked for the anesthesiologist. The second dream of pushing him out was taken from me when my baby decided presenting ass-first, breech, and pooping was the way to enter the world. The obstetrician recommended C-section for my safety and my baby's, but I will never know if that suggestion was genuine or based on race correction of the VBAC calculator.

Unfortunately, I never got another chance to push a bowling ball through my cooch. But even if I conceived again, I would still be unsure if my OB's advice that I forgo a trial of labor and go straight to C-section was informed by my race. And this is the particularly disturbing part. As a patient, I wouldn't be able to advocate for myself because chances are the OB would have said "because it's the safest plan for you and your baby," not "because Black women have primitive pelvises." Even the OB may not have been aware that this was the assumption of the VBAC calculator, but was simply trusting the validity of published research.

But getting back to the savagery. In 1943, while Nazi Germany was running concentration camps, American researchers were conducting a study of Black people with vitiligo, a disease in which patches of skin lose their color. They applied pain stimuli to pigmented and nonpigmented areas of skin "on the presumption that the increased pigmentation of the Negro's skin might account for the differences in the pain measurements."[14]

Although the barbaric experimentation eventually came to an end, the belief that Black people do not perceive pain lives on in Medicine today. In a 2016 study published by the National Academy of Sciences, roughly a third of White medical students and a quarter of White resident physicians surveyed believed Black people had thicker skin than White people; and about 7% and 4%, respectively, believed Black people's nerve endings were less sensitive than those of White people.[15]

Interestingly, in this same study, "Blacks have denser, stronger bones than whites" was among the statements about Black/White race differences that was considered true.[12] This belief in thicker skin and bones was used to justify the practice of using anywhere from 10% to 60% higher radiation doses in x-rays of Black people well into the 1960s, according to Bavli and Jones in a *New England Journal of Medicine* paper published in 2022.[16]

While small studies have shown a pattern of slightly higher bone density in Black people compared to White people, all failed to continue investigating to see whether specific factors such as how much weight-bearing exercise one did accounted for the differences. Interestingly, and by "interestingly" I mean racist af, they were content to just conclude these findings were based on inherent biological differences between Black and White people and generalize to all Black people.

In cardiology, the research is just as shaky. Many clinicians and laypersons alike may be familiar with the drug BiDil, the FDA-approved medication initially marketed to treat heart failure in Black people, but I'd imagine far fewer are aware that BiDil is a combination of isosorbide dinitrate and hydralazine—two ancient but generic medications that Medicine just repackaged as a capitalist marketing ploy. And still fewer people are aware that the whole idea was based upon old data spun into new data. In *Medical Apartheid,* Washington reports that the data claiming Black people died from heart failure at twice the rate of White people and justifying the need for a "Black pill" was not only old enough to legally drink had it been a person, but the disparity had already been resolved by interventions like improved access to medical care and lifestyle changes. The spinning, she went on, was in reporting that BiDil produced a 43% survival advantage in the African American Heart Failure Trial because 6.2% of participants who got the drug died, while 10.2% of those who didn't get the drug died. So while 6% is 40% lower than 10%, the absolute numbers aren't exactly jaw-dropping.

But it's really the teaching in medical training that several other commonly prescribed heart and blood pressure medications are said to *not* work in Black people that I doubt the vast majority are aware of—clinicians and the general public alike. As a fourth-year medical student, I remember reading in *Harrison's* pocket guide (a mini-version of the internist's bible) that beta blockers—a class of medication central to the treatment of heart failure—didn't work for Black people. Later, studies suggested that ACE inhibitors, another class of blood pressure medication central to treating heart failure and kidney disease with high urine protein, didn't work for Black people.[17] Up until the last few years, the popular evidence-based clinical reference UpToDate instructed me to consider evaluating patients for secondary causes for high blood pressure if they were under age 30 when their high blood pressure was diagnosed—but not if the person was Black. This recommendation has since been updated to "age less than 30 years in nonobese patients with a negative family history of hypertension and no other risk factors for hypertension," which is really no different since another section reports "Black race" as a risk factor for hypertension, another term for high blood pressure. Further, the latest version of the Joint National Committee report—the eighth, published in 2014—continued to endorse race-based hypertension treatment guidelines.[18]

Much of the rationale for why treating hypertension in Black people is particularly special is the "slavery hypertension hypothesis." The theory is that Black people have such high rates of difficult-to-control high blood pressure because only the Africans who survived the slave trade's Middle Passage were those with a genetic defect that prevented them from peeing out sodium. A body that holds on to extra sodium also holds on to extra water and, theoretically, is less likely to die of dehydration during the nearly three months it took to cross the Atlantic Ocean to the New World. So popular is this hypothesis, Oprah offered it as the "correct" answer on a May 2007 episode of her show when Dr. Mehmet Oz posed the question "Why so much high blood pressure among American Black people?"[19]

In 2020, I was part of a virtual panel discussion with a prominent Black cardiologist who supported it.

I pointed out that, in truth, it was just a hypothesis. Not one sliver of data to prove it, but "sounding good" passes for accepted science.

"Well, no one should be eating a high sodium diet anyway," he countered with only the slightest twinge of *how dare this bitch correct ME!* on his face.

No argument from me on that point, but what I take issue with is that instead of postulating that Black people had higher rates of hypertension because we continued recipes from enslaved ancestors accustomed to adding salt in order to make a pig's parts—from the rooter to the tooter—tasty, because that was all that was made available, Medicine would rather blame "African salt-retaining genes." Again, interesting.

And then there's pulmonology, Medicine's lung specialty. Here again we see the influence of Samuel Cartwright, who claimed his "research" showed that Black people's respiratory system functioned similar to "that of an infant child of the white race," thus showing "imperfect . . . vitalization of the blood in the lungs, as occurs in infancy, and a hebetude of torpor of intellect—from blood not sufficiently vitalized being distributed to the brain."[20] While being idle, says Cartwright, "the blood becomes so highly carbonized and deprived of oxygen, that it not only becomes unfit to stimulate the brain to energy, but unfit to stimulate the nerves of sensation distributed to the body." Therefore, he rationalized slave labor to be a good thing, which had positive physiological effects. To Cartwright, slave labor made Black people's "lungs perform the duty of vitalizing the blood more perfectly than is done when they are left free to indulge in idleness. It is the red, vital blood, sent to the brain, that liberates their mind when under the white man's control; and it is the want of a sufficiency of red, vital blood, that chains their mind to ignorance and barbarism, when in freedom."

Not long after English surgeon John Hutchinson's 1840 invention of the spirometer, a machine that can measure how much air a person inhales with a full breath and how quickly they can exhale that full breath, Cartwright built his own. He said that "the Negro has 20% smaller lungs than the White man" and someone asked, "How do you know this?" to which he replied, "because I measured it!" Nobody asked to see the measurements, much less question that any differences might be attributable to the fact that the enslaved were maintained in just enough shelter, food, and clothing necessary to work from "can't to can't"—can't see in the morning to can't see in the evening—except maybe on Sunday. Because of Jesus.

Race, as Lundy Braun asserts in her book on this topic, *Breathing Race into the Machine: The Surprising Career of the Spirometer from Plantation to Genetics*, was just built into the machine—ignoring measurable factors such as air pollution, which affects marginalized communities disproportionately, in establishing biological norms. Again, being Black is a good enough explanation.[21] So if the person doing the testing informs the machine software that analyzes the breathing measurements that the patient is Black, the report will be based on what is considered normal for a Black person. The first challenge to the accuracy of such "race adjustment" was effectively a doubling-down on the importance of race.

According to Esteban Burchard, a prominent pulmonology researcher, how Black one is matters. I met with him to try to understand his perspective.

He told me the story of a biracial patient he encountered, for context. The patient had suffered a toxic inhalation injury on the job and needed a spirometry test to show if he qualified for worker's compensation. The technician conducting the test assumed the patient was Black. But because the patient was only half Black, Burchard believed the adjustment for race was excessive and would, therefore, mean that the patient would have to be sicker than a White counterpart to qualify for worker's compensation. It was this encounter that served as the basis for his work to show that just how much African ancestry one has determines what "normal" lung capacity is.

In short, Burchard's work has attempted to answer my question for every "if Black" race correction: Exactly how Black does one need to be for this to apply?

This is supposedly answered through "ancestry informative markers," or AIMS—like a researcher's 23andMe. Burchard is not alone. Many researchers claim that ancestry is a more refined and specific alternative to race because ancestry estimates are inferred from objective informative markers in one's DNA, rather than by a simple racial yes/no. Problem is, these AIMS are based upon DNA samples from *living* people based upon the same continental origins—that is, European and African ancestry—that give rise to race. It stands to reason that a person with, say, 75% African ancestry markers would look quite different—and therefore probably be treated much differently by society—than someone with, say, just 25% African ancestry.

Nevertheless, Burchard claimed that quantifying "ancestry" improved accuracy for measuring lung volumes by 15%, and better predicted asthma severity compared to factors like air pollution and socioeconomic status. In a 2010 *New England Journal of Medicine* paper for which Burchard served as the senior author, the finding was that for every 1% increase in African ancestry, the lung volume decreased similarly.

This finding accounted for age, smoking, height, height squared, and body mass index (which is weight in kilograms divided by height squared).[22] Now, I'm just a little nephrologist, not a big-time pulmonologist or statistician, but this calculation seems to *over*-account for height, which essentially nullifies its effect. Furthermore, as another pulmonologist explained to me, one's sitting height is probably a better way to determine how big one's lungs ought to be, but sitting height has dropped out of research. Again, so interesting.

Even more interesting is anthropologist Duana Fullwiley's ethnographic account of how racial thinking persisted in Burchard's lab, published in *Social Studies of Science* in 2008.[23] She records a conversation in which data from a Puerto Rican population (a group known to have significant mixing of Native American, European, and African ancestry) suggested that European ancestry was higher in participants with asthma than those without asthma, and that African ancestry was associated with a better response to a frontline asthma medication—going against the original hypothesis "that Blacks were to blame," Burchard said, joking, looking at Fullwiley.

I asked Burchard how he thought of his research given the historical context, to which he responded: "These measurements have been going back a long time, at least to the 1850s. What people do with these measurements, I don't know the history of how some people might have used them to justify slavery, Nazis use measurement to justify racial purity. But that's neither here nor there, I'm not interested in the historical facts, I'm interested in the observed clinical observations that we have . . . I just try to stay away from the historical issues, I just look at the clinical differences. . . . So, I try to stay away from that political argument because I really just care about improving clinical diagnosis and accuracy of disease."

To suggest that one's research is somehow immune from society's interpretation is naïve at best. And if anybody should know this, it's Burchard, given that David Duke, former grand wizard of the Ku Klux Klan, has commended his work. But that's neither here nor there . . . I guess?

Burchard explained his own ancestry and family lineage as a means of justifying his work. Even pulled up an old image on his computer to prove it. Not so difficult, as it was part of a PowerPoint presentation he had recently given to medical students. Now, I never thought the stocky, tawny-colored man named Esteban was White, but it was important to him that he was not perceived as just some White guy talking about race. As if White people have a monopoly on anti-Blackness. And as if pointing out having 8% "African ancestry," as he did, wasn't so different from White folks pronouncing that because they had a Black friend/child/partner or whatever, they couldn't possibly be racist.

"You can see my great-grandfather is part African, he's got that n- [micro-pause] wavy hair." I'm trying to give the benefit of the doubt that the n-word he was able to hold back was "nappy," though that word coming from him would not have been much better.

Wait, there's more!

Cardiology also has the American Heart Association's Get with the Guide-lines Heart Failure Risk Score. Oncology has the Breast Cancer Surveillance Consortium Risk Calculator, the National Cancer Institute Breast Cancer Risk Assessment Tool, the Rectal Cancer Survival Calculator, *and* the Society of Thoracic Surgeons Short-Term Risk Calculator. Urology has the STONE Score. Rheumatology has the Osteoporosis Risk Score and the Fracture Risk Assessment Tool. Ophthalmology uses a different treatment protocol to treat Black people with glaucoma than White people. Even pediatrics has the Urinary Tract Infection Calculator for children.

They all include Black race as a factor in guiding clinician's decisions, and at the end of the day, each instance results in less desirable care for Black people—whether it be less surveillance for cancer, less evaluation for disease, less intensive care, or more potentially dangerous care.

What concerns me about all these attempts to prove that race is biological in general, and the Black race inferior in particular, is a common theme: Medicine's willingness to stop at race, rather than look for the "thing" that race is kinda, sorta associated with; Medicine's habit of only publishing what aligns with the assumption it already holds as truth; and Medicine's tendency to twist data so it sounds more absolute than it really is. That ain't science. And it's negligent.

CHAPTER 2

LOW-HANGING FRUIT

In the previous chapter, you may have noticed one glaring omission. I described the examples of race-based medicine in every specialty but one: nephrology, my specialty. You would be mistaken if you assumed that is because there are no examples. Rather, in terms of race-based medicine, nephrology has been doing the most. So much so that it has earned a chapter unto itself.

Nephrology, the study of kidney diseases, is arguably the medical specialty most egregious for assuming that Black people are inherently different from all other humans, but nobody said much about it for damn near 20 years. Because to Medicine, it just made sense that a Black person's kidneys would be inherently different.

Before 1999, the best way for doctors to estimate how well the kidneys were working—that is, how much blood could pass through the kidneys' tiny filters every minute of every day (the glomerular filtration rate, GFR)—was by requiring patients to collect a 24-hour sample of urine and have a blood test. They used this estimate to make critical medical decisions like proper dosing of medications, referring a patient to nephrology specialty care, and when to refer a patient for placement on the deceased donor kidney transplant waitlist. Not surprisingly, this test was considered cumbersome because, arguably, no patient relishes collecting their pee all day and storing it in their refrigerator alongside their milk and orange juice. Further, the urine collection was often off, less than or more than the full 24 hours, because patients would forget and flush their urine or misinterpret the instructions and collect too much. *Was I supposed to collect or flush my first pee this morning?*

But the landmark 1999 article in the *Annals of Internal Medicine* catchily titled "A More Accurate Method to Estimate Glomerular Filtration Rate from Serum Creatinine: A New Prediction Equation" changed all that.[1] All that was needed was a simple creatinine blood test to plug into an algebraic equation, then solve for *x*.

The equation was developed using the data of 197 Black and 1,304 White participants in the Modification of Diet in Renal Disease (MDRD) Study.[2] In their statistical analysis, researchers considered numerous *biological* variables—and self-reported Black or White race—as potential factors that might affect creatinine production or filtration. Of note, muscle mass was not directly measured. Rather, the equation was standardized for the average body size—based upon measurements of nine White Americans during the early 1910s, an average probably very different from the 1990s Americans in their study. That not-so-minor point aside, at the end of the equation's development, only three variables reportedly improved how close the estimation using creatinine came to replicating the "gold standard" (which requires a research lab, an IV, repeated blood draws, and essentially all day): age, sex, and Black race.

The analysis found that for a given creatinine, a Black person's estimated GFR was roughly 20% higher than a White person's. So a GFR of 20 for a White person is 24 for a Black person. This difference matters and—no exaggeration—can be the difference between living and dying.

Healthy kidneys can filter as much as 120 milliliters of blood every minute. Once the kidneys' filtering of blood drops below the threshold of 60 milliliters every minute, the kidneys can no longer fully function and do everything they are supposed to do—including making enough of the hormone that stimulates bone marrow to make blood and maintaining the blood's normal levels of minerals, like phosphorus, and electrolytes, like potassium. The kidneys also buffer all the acid in the food we eat. Yes, the kidneys do so much more than make urine. At an eGFR (estimated GFR) below 60, a person is defined as having moderate chronic kidney disease (CKD).

Once their GFR falls below 30, the person often needs specific medications to normalize blood levels. Some medications must be given in smaller doses or are no longer safe to use at all. A failure to make these adjustments may lead to harmful levels of medications in the body.

At a GFR of 20, a patient can be referred for kidney transplant evaluation and placed on the waitlist to get a kidney from a deceased donor. The amount of time on the waitlist is one of the most important factors determining when someone can get a deceased donor kidney—which can take anywhere between 3 and 10 years, depending on factors like where you live and your blood type. Some people accrue enough time on the waitlist that they get what is called a preemptive transplant, meaning they never have to endure dialysis. Most people will need some form of kidney replacement (dialysis or transplant) by a GFR of 5. Without it, a person may die within a little over a week to a few months, depending upon various factors.

For some people *years* can pass before the GFR falls from 24 to 20. People with GFR in or below this range lose muscle mass, so assuming someone's kidney function is 20% higher than others simply because they are Black is particularly problematic. It's problematic because far more people are waiting for a kidney than kidneys are available—with 13 people on the waitlist *dying* every day while waiting for a kidney. So a 20% difference based on being Black alone matters.

Researchers offered no rationale for why or how being Black affects how much creatinine a body produces, nor did they explain how being Black affects how the kidneys filter creatinine—even though proposing a plausible reason for why thing X might affect thing Y is a basic tenet of research and, therefore, should be accounted for. Lacking a plausible explanation to reassure that statistically significant findings aren't just by chance is analogous to throwing wads of chewed gum against a wall and seeing what sticks.

Instead, the researchers attempted to explain their statistically significant result after the fact, stating that "Black persons have higher muscle mass than White persons," as supposedly supported by three small studies they cited. None of the studies had much, if anything, to do with muscle mass, nor were the three studies substantial enough to warrant generalization to an entire population. A small study by Harsha and colleagues published in 1978 found 99 Black children had slightly less body fat than 143 White children.[3] A smaller study by Cohn and colleagues published in 1977 found 47 Black men and women had slightly higher total-body potassium, which the authors postulated would be important in determining skeletal mass, than "normal" White people of similar age and gender.[4] An even smaller study by Worrall and colleagues published in 1990 found racial variation in creatine kinase of 30 Black and 30 White participants was independent of lean body mass (muscles, bones, and body fluids).[5] Furthermore, one can trace the Harsha study back to the pseudo-science of the 1800s directly because, as they cited, "systematic anthropometric differences between the races have long been recognized."[6]

Nevertheless, Medicine concluded *all* Black people had higher muscle mass than all White people—from a study with 197 Black people. Based upon what is published, it occurred to no one that the reason why accounting for race better aligned with the gold standard GFR in a Black and a White participant with the same creatinine was because more Black people in the study had diabetes (which is known to cause higher GFR at a given creatinine) and high blood pressure (which along with diabetes accounts for two-thirds of chronic kidney disease in the US) than the White participants—and not because "Black people's kidneys are different."

This conclusion was carried into the development of an even more precise creatinine-based equation from the Chronic Kidney Disease Epidemiology Collaboration (CKD-EPI).[7] Published in 2009, the manuscript revealed that not only was the continued use of Black race as a variable in the CKD-EPI equation not questioned, but the researchers took it one step further. In a study population of nearly 10,000 where there was a smattering of diversity, with 5% of the participants identified as Asian and Hispanic, the researchers *decided* to include a race variable defined as Black versus Other at the start of equation development, effectively implying that Black people were the "other," biologically distinct from *all* other humans.[8]

Medicine even tried to "other" Black people in the development of an equation based upon cystatin C, a small protein produced at a constant rate by all nucleated cells that can be measured with a blood test and is less problematic than creatinine. Unlike creatinine, cystatin C is not affected by muscle mass and is more accurate than creatinine in estimating GFR. In the 2012 *New England Journal of Medicine* paper explaining how the equation was developed, however, we learned that yet again researchers considered race as a possible factor in predicting measured GFR and offered no rationale for why a protein found in all nucleated cells might be higher or lower or filtered differently in Black people and Black people alone.[9] Perhaps we have Jesus, Buddha, Allah, Jehovah, Mama Earth, and all 10,000 Hindu gods to thank that the statistics didn't support that bullshit.

It wasn't until 2005 that some labs started doing the math for clinicians by reporting two numbers: the estimated GFR and the estimated GFR "if African American" based upon the 1999 MDRD equation. Having finished medical school before this equation was published, I wasn't aware of it or its origin until I started my nephrology fellowship in 2007.

Unlike my peers who had lived and breathed everything kidney for much of their residency training, which had just ended the week before, I was new to nephrology and had been a primary care doctor and researcher since completing my residency training five years prior. I went into nephrology because I wanted to do research that would inform eliminating racial differences in access to kidney transplants after a nephrologist told me doing so would elevate my research and how it was perceived when I was just looking for a project. Everything else in nephrology, including equations to estimate kidney function, was uncharted territory for me.

In that first week of fellowship, before we fellows would be tossed into the deep end of patient care and suddenly expected to be a "specialist" in all things kidney, the fellowship director gave my five non-Black peers and me an orientation. One of the lectures was regarding equations to estimate kidney function.

He explained that the multiplier for "if African American" race was intended as a proxy for muscle mass. That Black race was being used as a shortcut for assessing muscle mass immediately struck me as extremely odd—and racist.

"But what about the petite Black woman or the frail old Black person?" I asked the fellowship director. "Wouldn't the assumption be wrong for them?"

"You raise a good point," the fellowship director nodded, pausing briefly before moving on to his next PowerPoint slide, the academic version of *anyhoo*. The conversation was done, and it seemed I was the only one who took issue with the multiplier for "if African American."

I didn't bring it up again until months later when fellows were invited to have one-on-one meetings with Andrew Levey, the lead author of the equation development paper, himself. He was the quintessential doctor. An average-looking, average-built White man with gray hair and glasses. I smiled and said hello when I entered the conference room where he had waited for each fellow, and I took my seat in the chair on the side of the conference table perpendicular to his.

I opened our one-on-one by letting him know that we had kidney donation in common. He had indirectly donated a kidney to his wife: one of those swap agreements in which two people wanted to donate to their loved one but couldn't because of something like incompatible blood types, so they each gave their kidney to the other person's loved one. "How does it feel to be a hero?" he asked.

I could tell by his puffed-out chest and the smirk on his face that it was more of a serious "welcome to the club" statement than a question. Not to border on man-hating, but I thought it was just like a man to call himself a hero after donating a kidney. Like getting yourself a "Best Person Ever" mug after you mowed your octogenarian neighbor's lawn.

I turned the conversation to the eGFR equations. "Did you all consider the impact of using race as a proxy for muscle mass?" I asked.

His eyes stretched as he seemingly searched for an answer. "Well, clinicians have to use their judgment when interpreting the result," he said.

"But how would clinicians know how to use their judgment if they don't know race is supposed to be a proxy for muscle mass?" I pushed back.

In response, he lifted his arm and turned his wrist to look at his watch in the grandest body language of *How much longer do I have to meet with this bitch?* I'd ever seen in my life. I took the not-so-subtle hint and changed the conversation to the topic of my research.

I didn't bring up the subject again until I had completed the fellowship and joined the faculty roughly 18 months later as a full-fledged attending nephrologist, someone who resident physicians and medical students would come to see in clinic as part of their training. After the residents and medical students saw a patient, I would sit down with them to discuss the case and do a little teaching about nephrology. I used these opportunities to educate them, one by one, about why Black is used in our equations and why it was important to look beyond the race of the person in front of them. Some of these young and wannabe doctors had wondered about the origin of race correction, but none knew why or how it came to be used.

Still, my colleagues were dismissive, and it wasn't until I was writing my first book, *Hundreds of Interlaced Fingers*, in late 2015 that I happened upon University of Pennsylvania law professor Dorothy Roberts's TEDMED Talk.[10] In it, she discussed the issue of "race correction" from her perspective as a biracial, Black-identifying person. I felt validated and fortified enough to include it in my book and my TEDx San Francisco Talk in 2017. Two years later, I was among the group of doctors, including family medicine and laboratory medicine colleagues, reprimanded for removing "if African American" from GFR reporting in our electronic medical record at San Francisco General Hospital. Those reprimanding me were my boss, the chief of nephrology, and Neil Powe, the chair of medicine, making him the boss of my boss. Powe, a prominent Black internist who had been doing research in chronic kidney disease for so long that even nephrologists forget he was not a nephrologist, had also been my research mentor for the last decade.

"You all should leave this to the experts," Powe said condescendingly. As if our family medicine colleagues weren't smart enough to have an opinion and didn't deserve his respect. As if I wasn't a highfalutin program-trained board-certified nephrologist—and as if he was. It had not occurred to me that I would have to argue to eliminate a racist equation with Powe, a Black man in Medicine.

"I know Andy personally," he said, name-dropping Levey, the physician researcher leading equation development.

I was not impressed.

"The world was a different place 30 years ago," he went on, as if that was supposed to justify the continuation of race-based reporting and the inclusion of race in the first place.

Now, I do not presume to understand or judge what Black men in their early sixties who have achieved great academic success and stature have had to endure, swallow, and ignore in order to be successful. But through Powe's reaction I realized how deeply the patriarchy and White supremacy are ingrained in Medicine. Previously, I had believed that if a Black person had been at the equation development table, race would have never been included as something to be "corrected" for. But after that day, I was reminded that all skin folk ain't kin folk. Powe became the Clarence Thomas of Medicine for me.

Furthermore, it was the so-called experts who had created the issue nearly 20 years prior and perceived no need for change, so leaving it to them was not an option. Still, the conversation didn't gain real traction until the medical students got involved.

Now, back in my medical school days, which were right after they made medical students walk uphill through the snow both ways to get to class but before social media, nobody asked how you felt about your training. If anything, speaking without being spoken to was aggressively discouraged.

But they raise medical students differently these days. The opinions of medical students are sought out, and speaking up seems to be applauded, at least until they hit the clinical wards in their third year. As a result, when second-year students felt the curriculum was designed to teach them to be racist rather than the conscious, caring doctors they hoped to be for their future patients regardless of race, they mounted a protest. Through social media, petitions, and presentations, medical students spearheaded the effort that *forced* a national conversation.

Some wondered why we were all making such a big deal about it. They doubted the equation developers set out to be overtly racist or had malintent. For the most part, I agree. I believe most clinicians and medical researchers strive to do the right thing. However, we all exist within a society plagued by structural racism to which none of us is immune. So it doesn't really matter the intention of the equation developers. After all, as they say, the path to Hell is paved with good intentions. What mattered was the existence of a "race correction" that had harmful consequences for Black people.

Most of Medicine's nephrologists, and those entrenched in kidney-related research, were the staunchest of critics. The vast majority of nephrologists have been most resistant to the idea of eliminating the race multiplier, which is astounding in a specialty that prides itself on precision. There are equations to calculate solute deficit, excess, and fractional excretions; dialysis adequacy; appropriate acute and chronic respiratory responses for metabolic acid-base disturbances; the likelihood of advancing to end-stage kidney disease; and the likelihood of dying within six months of starting dialysis—often to two decimal points. Basic scientists have elucidated ion channels and dozens upon dozens of genetic mutations responsible for disease throughout the nephron. But when it comes to race, it doesn't seem to matter if one is 51%, 78%, or 22.56% African American—a simple yes or no appears to be all the precision we need in the United States, while the United Kingdom has decided that 51% is the cutoff—a biracial person is considered "not African American" in eGFR interpretation. And in the 20 years since publication of the original article codifying race correction, there had been no efforts to determine what "Black race" is actually measuring. It was at best akin to finding that carrying a lighter or matches is associated with lung cancer while never considering that cigarettes, or more precisely, identifying the specific carcinogens within cigarettes, are the true independent predictors of lung cancer.

Medicine shouted a myriad of hyperbolic—and unproven—negative consequences of dropping race correction with their entire chest, because it would make Black people's kidney function look worse, thus leading to all kinds of disasters. Medications would be denied to Black people, they claimed. Research would be impeded! Kidney donation would be thwarted! Black people's anxiety would be provoked, and their life insurance applications denied! Besides, they insisted, dropping race correction won't eliminate the racial disparities in kidney disease—like the fact that Black people reach kidney failure nearly four times faster than White people. Hell, they warned, racial disparities in health outcomes might even be aggravated!

Mind you, all of these predictions rested upon the assumption that the evidence supporting race correction was actually valid. And they completely ignored the actual negative consequences of race correction for 20 years. Furthermore, none of the critics seemed to be moved by the fact that "race correction" did not improve estimating GFR in several African nations—including West African nations where most American Black people are assumed to originate from because of American chattel slavery. Even Levey himself wrote a commentary acknowledging that race correction wasn't necessary, perhaps because of "dietary factors." Yet in American Medicine, it remained all about Black race.

As a result, it took a whole-ass task force from two leading organizations in the US dedicated to preventing, treating, and, hopefully, one day, curing kidney disease: the American Society of Nephrology and the National Kidney Foundation. The task force selected various health professionals and patients, including "individuals with expertise in diagnosis, management, and treatment of kidney disease; measurement and estimation of GFR; health care disparities; epidemiology and clinical research; laboratory medicine; pharmacy; health services research; patient safety; patient experience with care; patient quality of life; medical education; and prevention/public health."[11] Cynthia Delgado—a Latina and my nephrology co-fellow who chose to point out how "diverse" we, a class of five Asians and the two of us, already were when I pressed the fellowship director for more Black and Hispanic fellows—and Neil Powe served as co-chairs.

I was not invited to serve on the task force.

After two years of I don't know how many hours of extensive delibera-tion and testimony to decide if the race multiplier—the thing that had been inserted without any valid evidence or debate—should remain, the task force's final consensus was what some of us had always known: estimating equations for kidney function should *not* include race. Ultimately, a new creatinine-based equation pooling all the data from the CKD-EPI equation was released, as well as a recommendation to use the cystatin C–based equation for situations where more accuracy might influence clinical decisions.[12]

When I reflect, I realize my initial astonishment at how much it would take to stop "race correction" was unwarranted. Still, disappointment was merited for sure, disappointment that it took nearly 20 years to assemble a task force and another eight months for that task force to come to the obvious decision. In the quest to divorce all medical specialties from the notion that race has bio-logical meaning beyond superficial groupings around skin color, hair texture, and facial features, removing race from GFR estimation was supposed to be the low-hanging fruit—easy pickings, because a fully vetted and *better* alternative to creatinine in cystatin C already existed. Instead, the Establishment fixated on cystatin C being unvalidated and 5 to 10 times more expensive than creati-nine, completely ignoring that creatinine was not validated across labs around the country until the early 2000s and the reported cost of cystatin C reflected having to send samples to be run by an outside lab at the time. Laboratory physicians at San Francisco General Hospital estimated that even with the cost difference, about fivefold at the time, it would only amount to $60,000 per year if everybody switched to ordering cystatin C as often as creatinine. I'd imagine the hospital's paper towel budget was more than that. Plus, the cost would undoubtedly come down once the lab learned how to run it in-house.

But, certainly, astonishment ought to be reserved for someone acting out of character. Medicine trying to disregard anything that challenged its com-mitment to White supremacy was par for the course. To deny the status quo would mean reevaluating the appropriateness of *all* past recommendations and *all* study conclusions that informed drug approval, kidney disease prognosis, and funding. It might even mean admitting that a bunch of students and "non-experts" were right all along: It was never appropriate to include race in the development of GFR estimating equations. I could count on one hand the number of nephrologists who supported removing race correction from the start, and I have yet to hear a critic acknowledge that they were on the wrong side of that particular history. Instead, they try to pretend it was their idea all along. "The issue is a moral issue," said Powe in a September 2021 article in *The New York Times*. "It is time to remove race from the equation."[13]

Sadly, nephrology's bullshit doesn't even end here. Nephrology also has the Kidney Donor Risk Index, which suggests kidneys from dead Black people won't last as long as kidneys from all other races of dead folks. This is based upon another one of Medicine's overgeneralizations about APOL1, a gene associated with kidney failure. Like sickle cell disease, it's thought that evolution created a couple of variations in this gene (variants) to protect people from sleeping sickness, a highly deadly disease spread by the tsetse fly and mostly confined to sub-Saharan Africa. Inheriting one variant from a parent protects a person from sleeping sickness, but getting a copy from each parent creates a much higher risk of high blood pressure-related kidney failure compared to people with no variants. Just having one variant will increase a person's risk of this kind of kidney failure. High blood pressure accounts for about 20% of kidney failure, second only to diabetes.

Medicine behaves as if *only* Black people can have an APOL1 variant; that *every* Black person has two variants; and that *everybody* with two variants is going to have kidney failure—which is not even close to reality. In truth, the variants are most often found among people of West African descent, but are also found among European American, Pakistani, and Latin American groups. Further, only about 20 of every 100 Black Americans have one variant, and 13 of every 100 Black Americans have two variants.[14] Further, about 2 of every 100 people with no variants, 4 of every 100 people with one variant, and 12 of every 100 people with two variants will develop kidney failure in their lifetime.

So not all Black people, or even the majority, will develop kidney failure. To put it another way, only a sliver of a sliver of a sliver of Black folks will.

The problem with overgeneralization was shown in a study published in the *American Journal of Transplantation* in 2017.[15] Researchers found that when they actually tested for APOL1—a test that can be done in the same amount of time it takes to get results for other routinely checked labs like HIV and hepatitis C—transplant centers were *wrong* about decisions to throw away kidneys from dead Black people *85% of the time*. This is particularly ridiculous when one considers that an estimated 13 people die every day while waiting for a donor kidney.

Currently, patients awaiting a deceased donor kidney get to decide if they prefer a standard criteria donor kidney or an expanded criteria donor kidney. The standard criteria donor kidney is considered pretty much perfect, while the expanded criteria donor kidney is . . . not. Maybe the donor was a little older, had some high blood pressure, had slightly elevated creatinine, or died of a stroke. The bottom line is that an expanded criteria kidney is believed to have fewer pees left than the standard kidney. But on average, "not so perfect" comes along more often than pristine, meaning a shorter wait time for the potential recipient. If I'm 45 and healthy aside from my failed kidneys, I would be willing to wait the extra years for a perfect kidney. But if I'm, say, 70, diabetic, and already on dialysis, then not so perfect is probably good enough for me and the number of pees I'll need to take until the end of my life. Where would a kidney from a Black donor fit in? How many people would rather take their chances of dying while waiting for a donor kidney than accept one from a Black donor?

It's the Medicine breeding anti-Blackness, for me.

CHAPTER 3

THE SEARCH CONTINUES

One would think that after the second wave of debunking race science as pseudoscience, we would be past teasing biological meaning from race. While there have been some efforts to remove race from clinical algorithms, a contingent can't seem to break from the past. I'm not talking about some random internet troll making up statistics or even an obscure little makeshift journal surreptitiously backed by the KKK. I'm talking about *peer-reviewed* articles published in top medical journals by major medical societies.

On September 28, 2021, I listened to my colleague Raymond Givens give a virtual lecture about race in Medicine. As one must when you're lecturing to an audience less engrossed in a topic than yourself, Givens started with a lot of background "let's get on the same page" content. And while I recognized it as necessary, having to enlighten a predominantly White audience on such Racism 101 topics like redlining and segregation is symptomatic of the willful ignorance that keeps us from getting to the part where we discuss what needs to happen next. (One could argue this is exactly what is happening in this book, but at least I'm not constrained by a defined time. The reader just needs to hang in there until the last chapter to find out what we demonstrably can do and must do to combat the bullshit next.)

But I perked up when he used an article published a year earlier in the *Journal of the American Medical Association* (*JAMA*)—one of the top medical journals in the world—titled "Racial/Ethnic Variation in Nasal Gene Expression of Transmembrane Serine Protease 2 (TMPRSS2)" as an example of how researchers ignore basic logic to link race to a genetic predisposition to disease.[1] In this research letter, Bunyavanich and colleagues included a figure showing that, in their study, Black people had markedly higher levels of the nasal gene than White, Latinx, and Asian people. They intimated that this higher gene expression may explain why Black people were contracting COVID disproportionately.

Givens pointed out the flaws in the researchers' logic. They suggested higher expression mattered when nobody had shown the biological pathway between expression and COVID. They had tried to sell the importance of the gene by comparing it to a study that found lower gene activity in the prostate tissue of Black men with prostate cancer compared to White men. (If this sounds convoluted, that's because it is. A reach if I ever saw one.) They didn't explain why the expressions in samples from Latinx people were similar to those from White people yet had much higher rates of COVID infection. Now, all of this may be attributable to a system that rewards individuals for their sheer number of publications, rather than quality research and writing, thus incentivizing writing five nuanced papers when one comprehensive paper would have sufficed. But it also underscores how any suggestion that Black people have worse health outcomes than everybody else overall not due to racism, or systematic oppression, but rather their genetic predisposition to disease, is instantly publishable even if it doesn't make logical sense.

Oops, *JAMA* did it again in 2023 with Vart and colleagues' "Effectiveness and Safety of Dapagliflozin for Black and White Patients with Chronic Kidney Disease in North and South America: A Secondary Analysis of a Randomized Controlled Trial."[2] If ever there was an automatic pass in academic medicine, it's with the words "randomized controlled trial." Researchers and readers alike behave as if a study that assigns people to treatment A or treatment B, like the flip of a coin, is automatically free of human bias (and that any study that is not randomized and controlled is basically trash). Even if that were the case, in the end, humans injecting meaning into the findings can wash all that objectivity out. The first clue that this was the case for Vart and colleagues' research letter is that it is a secondary analysis, meaning they didn't set up the study to find an answer to this particular question. That it was a research letter (limited to 600 words) and not a full article (up to 3,000 words) is another clue they didn't have much to say. The main study was to see if dapagliflozin, a sodium-glucose cotransporter-2 (SGLT2) inhibitor, one of the latest classes of drugs to treat diabetes, was better at preventing worsening kidney disease and cardiovascular events in patients who already had chronic kidney disease (and therefore already at risk of these negative outcomes) than taking a pill that just looked like dapagliflozin, that is, a placebo. To look at differences by race is that same old bullshit the paper's authors decided to do because, as they originally asserted, "Black and White patients experience a distinct array of comorbid conditions and can respond differently to interventions."[3]

At face value, this statement implies there is some biological difference between Black and White people. To paraphrase the researchers, Black people don't even get the same diseases as White people, and even if they did, the same medications won't work for them. The "proof" used to back up this assertion was two citations. The first citation, a 2008 publication by Adler and Rehkopf, is about racial health disparities and how poverty contributes to the disparities.[4] The second citation was a 2001 editorial entitled "Racial Differences in the Response to Drugs—Pointers to Genetic Differences" by A. J. Wood in the *New England Journal of Medicine* touting two studies in the same issue that supposedly addressed the effect of race on important drugs used in heart failure, which would "help physicians choose the best therapy for heart failure patients of different races."[5] But in truth, another article (Yancy and colleagues) found that carvedilol (a beta blocker) was equally effective for Black and non-Black people with heart failure.[6] A different article (Exner and colleagues) did find that Black patients treated with enalapril (an angiotensin-converting enzyme, or ACE, inhibitor) didn't experience the same reduction in risk for hospitalization for heart failure that White patients did.[7] Never mind that the Black patients in the study were far less likely to be college educated and much more likely to have experienced "financial distress" in the past year compared to their White counterparts. Still, in his writing, Wood argues that a genetic difference must be at hand because another group of researchers found that the frequency of a specific enzyme that affects drug metabolism (specifically CYP2D6 variants) is high in "Black Americans and Africans . . . but virtually absent from White and Asian populations." I get it. When one starts throwing in genetic markers and frequencies, it sounds legitimate. But "high" in this case is not over 34%, and "virtually absent" ain't zero, and to pretend any of it can explain why Black people die younger and more often than White people, instead of, say, the various forms of racism they endure, is nonsensical. But instead of making this argument, we tend to get into a *how do you explain this* type of discussion every time someone questions this assertion.

I'm reminded of the peer review process for my article "Let's Stop Playing the Race Card."[8] One reviewer wrote, "Lastly, the author states that we may be too willing to equate race with genetic meaning but fails to cite other notable studies which show racial differences presumably secondary to genetic polymorphisms," and offered Camille Powe and colleagues' article "Vitamin D-Binding Protein and Vitamin D Status of Black Americans and White Americans" published in 2013 in the *New England Journal of Medicine*—the top-ranking medical journal—as an example.[9] Indeed, this study displays convincing data and graphics demonstrating that in a population of Black and White people, Black participants had a more frequent genetic variation coinciding with lower levels of vitamin D and vitamin D-binding protein than White participants, suggesting that the amount of free vitamin D (not attached to the binding protein) was similar, thus making the point that we are perhaps overdiagnosing and overtreating vitamin D deficiency in Black people. But what is troubling is that the researchers equate the genetic variation with race, with only one phrase buried in the "Discussion" section acknowledging that skin pigmentation may have had something to do with the numbers. It is a different thing to say "Black people have X and Y" and not "More darkly pigmented people have X and Y," because, indeed, not all Black people are dark-skinned and not all dark-skinned people are Black.

Still, Vart and colleagues use this logic to go on to state, "Black patients are more likely to develop salt-sensitive hypertension, less responsive to renin-angiotensin-aldosterone system inhibitors, and nearly 4-fold more likely to develop progressive chronic kidney disease (CKD), leading to kidney failure," to justify the importance of their analysis. Because "it is unclear whether the effectiveness and safety of SGLT2 inhibitors differ between Black and White patients with CKD." No matter that they were conflating unproven biological hypotheses and faulty research with societal realities.

But this is how it goes; researchers cite articles that place too much weight on their suspect findings by citing another article that made an assertion that is, at best, two degrees of separation from a study completely steeped in pseudoscience. This happens continually because people tend not to read the details or question findings that agree with their worldview. Even people in Medicine.

"So, are we to just ignore the findings of major studies like the Antihypertensive and Lipid-Lowering Treatment to Prevent Heart Attack Trial (ALLHAT)?" I've heard people ask. If the study makes pronouncements of what does and doesn't work for Black people, then hell yes. But let me further tell you why, as explained through a tweetorial (who said social media can't be educational?) originally posted by Anjana Sharma, a family medicine physician and researcher, in 2019. Sharma credits the senior family medicine resident physician at the time, Adeola Oni-Orisan, who presented the study's details as part of a journal club when she was an intern.

ALLHAT was a randomized, double-blind (neither the researcher nor the patient knew which drug they were taking), controlled trial of more than 40,000 people aged 55 and older who had hypertension and at least one other risk factor for coronary heart disease (like diabetes or a prior heart attack), conducted at over 600 centers around North America.[10] The participants were to take chlorthalidone (a diuretic), amlodipine (a calcium channel blocker), lisinopril (an ACE inhibitor), or doxazosin (an alpha blocker that was abandoned early on) plus second- or third-tier medications to get their blood pressure controlled and see if one was better at preventing heart attacks and a slew of other bad outcomes like dying of anything or having a stroke. The trial was conducted from February 1994 through March 2002 and findings were published in *JAMA* in December 2002. Impressive, I know, so why wouldn't we trust everything that came from it?[11]

As Sharma's tweetorial explained, the main finding was that there were no major differences between the three drugs in preventing the primary outcome of heart attacks. Duh, because one doesn't need to know much about these medications to doubt any of them could prevent a heart attack. This is why all the attention went to subgroup analyses—analyses among groups within the larger study with a shared characteristic, such as race or gender.

Now, there's nothing inherently wrong with subgroup analyses per se. Why spend all that time and taxpayer money asking and answering only one question? That would be a waste. However, researchers must be careful about how much is read into findings that a study wasn't based on. When looking at studies, researchers must consider if the number of people included was enough and if the duration of the study itself was long enough to detect a difference in an outcome—outcomes that are noticeably different from what occurs in typical reality. The chances of seeing something that isn't true is about 1 in 20, so when slicing and dicing data dozens of different ways and throwing them against the wall, something is bound to stick, even if it's not true. It could simply be by chance. That's why we should start with a plausible explanation or hypothesis for why we think the thing we're testing for might be true. Hint: "'cuz they Black" is not good enough.

In subanalyses, they found that chlorthalidone was better than amlodipine for preventing heart failure and better than lisinopril for preventing coronary artery disease, stroke, and heart failure. That's all fine and unproblematic, but then the researchers go on to look at it all by race and find that the Black folks who needed second- and third-tier medications to get their blood pressure under control were at slightly higher risk for stroke if they were taking lisinopril instead of amlodipine. And like a kids' game of telephone, one finding out of dozens of "no difference" findings about stroke risk went to "Black people should be treated with calcium channel blockers" and fueled the "ACE inhibitors don't work for Black people" fire, even though we know ACE inhibitors are cornerstones of heart failure treatment and, for folks with high protein in their urine, kidney protective. This misinformation has been going on for 20 years and counting.

But even before I went down the rabbit hole on the Vart research letter, I took to Twitter and quote-tweeted the article. Minus the abbreviations and hashtags induced by Twitter character limit and view-boosting efforts, I tweeted: "Race-based medicine persists because journals keep publishing it. Another article with old, unproven hypotheses about Black people to justify the study with no mention of structural racism as a potential reason for observed differences. Editors must require better."

By no means did that tweet go viral, but it did get noticed by some key people, at least by *JAMA*'s editor-in-chief and my prior research mentor Kirsten Bibbins-Domingo who direct messaged me telling me so. Soon after, an apology editorial was written, and the authors revised the paper's introduction. Sadly, but not unexpectedly, both were some bullshit. I say the apology was insincere because the editors started well, acknowledging the harm caused and accepting responsibility, but devolved into full-on excusing behavior in an attempt to explain away the error: *See, what had happened was* the descriptive framework that the authors included in the original submission was deleted to accommodate a reviewer's suggestion to shorten the "Introduction" (yes, they really tried to pin it on a reviewer). It would have been so much better had they simply acknowledged the more plausible explanation: An article passed through multiple iterations with at least three peer reviewers and at least three editors before publication because none of them saw any issues with it. Because people tend not to question, much less scratch below the surface of or attempt to dig deeper into, anything that agrees with their perceived notions of how the world works, especially regarding race. Medicine is no exception.

The revamped article was somehow worse, attempting gymnastics even Simone Biles wouldn't try. The republished article read: "Relative to White patients, Black patients in North and South America often experience obstacles in accessing high-quality health care, including structural racism, and, in general, experience a distinct array of comorbid conditions and social determinants of health that can affect longevity, disease trajectory, health-related quality of life, and response to therapeutic interventions."[12] But get this: They cited the Adler paper again but replaced the citation for Wood's editorial with, interestingly, an opposing editorial—"Racial Profiling in Medical Research" by R. S. Schwartz—in the same issue to support their new contrived rationale.[13] Schwartz makes the same arguments I make here—that race is some shit colonizers made up, and any attempt to equate that made-up shit with biology is pseudoscience (sure, he said it in a more *New England Journal*–like way). Yet according to the authors, the distinct array of comorbid conditions was still due to the same line about Black people and salt-sensitive hypertension blah blah blah, which they repeated verbatim. It was still important to do the analysis "because of previously reported differences in experiences regarding comorbidities, barriers to care, and social determinants of health, there could be differences in reported findings of effectiveness and safety of SGLT2 inhibitors among Black and White patients with CKD."

If I'm being gracious, I'd offer that at least the editors and researchers attempted to twist themselves into some semblance of making it right. But I'm not feeling gracious, because these issues persist after debunking pseudoscience, and so-called racial reckonings are simply negligent toward Black people. After all the twisting and flipping, dapagliflozin worked for both Black and White patients alike. Go figure.

Some researchers have attempted to evolve from these simple Black-White comparisons to suggest a genetic basis by quantifying just how Black or White someone is. They determine this by determining exactly how much African or European ancestry a person has, based on DNA markers from living reference populations classified by race, ethnicity, or nationality. How can one call living folks ancestors? Using ancestry to classify race in an attempt to be more precise is no better than putting lipstick on the proverbial pig. It's still "race." They just tried to get fancy with it.

I formed a writing team with Dr. Amy Non, a genetic anthropologist, and Dr. Jessica Cerdeña, a biocultural and medical anthropologist turned medical student, to explain why. Together we coauthored three perspective/viewpoint papers, all published in 2022: "Racialising Genetic Risk: Assumptions, Realities and Recommendations" for *The Lancet* (one of the world's oldest and highest-impact journals, founded in England, hence the spelling of *racializing*). Then we wrote "Genomic Supremacy: The Harm of Conflating Genetic Ancestry and Race" for the lesser well-known *Human Genomics* journal (after nine rejections). Lastly, we wrote my personal favorite, "The Misuse of Race in the Search for Disease-Causing Alleles" for The Art of Medicine, a special section in *The Lancet*.[14]

The Art of Medicine paper is my favorite, not just because I took the lead. In medical academia, the order in which coauthors appear on a paper means something. The last author is the most senior in the subject matter and has the final say on when a paper is ready to be submitted for journal review. The first author is the one who dreamed up the idea for the project and does the lion's share of the work. On papers with many coauthors, the amount and kind of contributions can vary from offering significant edits to barely earning the ink it takes to print one's name. After the second author, being a "middle author" does little more than pad one's total number of publications for promotion, which is why people do it.

For our first two papers, I earned my second authorship by largely functioning as the "regular-people language translator" and "reviewer heavy" (both important roles to temper the uber-expert speak so academic non-anthropologists like myself could understand the content and quell authors' tendency to obsequiously thank asshole peer reviewers for their "insightful" comments for fear of having a paper rejected behind bruised egos), but leading the Art of Medicine paper allowed me to flex my artistic muscles. I was a successful-enough scientific research writer to earn a promotion from assistant to associate professor before leaving the academic world. Yet the formulaic structure with the evergreen and inconsequential "more research is needed" conclusion is not nearly as satisfying as writing for the people. What I took as the highest compliment for my first book,

Hundreds of Interlaced Fingers, was that it read like a novel. Impressive since I had to explain the kidneys on a molecular level without putting the reader to sleep!

For "The Misuse of Race in the Search for Disease-Causing Alleles" paper, I had the brilliant idea (if I do say myself) to build upon the seminal work of Dr. Camara Jones, "Levels of Racism: A Theoretic Framework and a Gardener's Tale," published in the *American Journal of Public Health* in 2000.[15] Jones used allegory to help the reader understand racism on three levels: institutionalized, personally mediated, and internalized.

Her allegory goes like this: The gardener (i.e., the government) has two flower boxes. She knows that one flower box is filled with rich, fertile soil and the other with poor, rocky soil. She has two packets of seeds. One will bear plants with red blossoms, the other pink. She prefers red over pink, so she plants the red-blossoming seeds in the rich soil and the pink-blossoming seeds in the poor soil because she doesn't like pink blossoms enough to take her ass to the store and get some more good soil (i.e., institutionalized racism). She dislikes the pink blossoms so much that when the wind blows some pink seeds into the red flower box, she plucks them out before they can establish themselves (i.e., personally mediated racism). Of course, over the years the red-blossoming plants grow big and beautiful in their rich soil, while the pink-blossoming plants are scrawny and ugly. This only reinforces the gardener's belief system: red-blossoming plants are better than pink-blossoming ones. The pink-blossoming plants are so scrawny and ugly that some eventually start to hate themselves. They hate themselves so much so that if the bees try to pollinate them, they scream at the bees. "Don't bring us any of that pink pollen!" They, too, prefer red—i.e., internalized racism, where the red-blossoming plants represent Whiteness and the pink-blossoming plants are Black people (and to lesser degrees every other marginalized group, because at least they ain't Black). We see this in Black people lifting up (and possibly making up) non-Black ancestors. Cherokee Indian is a popular one. Blackfoot is probably a close second. And then there's the claiming of nationalities—German, Irish, French. Anything to keep from being all Black, as if they aren't all White, and the common denominator for all of them wasn't slavery. They all owned, bought, sold, and raped us, but some of us are just proud to say they aren't all Black.

So my writing group took Jones's allegory further, to highlight how theories and beliefs about race having biological meaning have created a legacy of bullshit that has real implications for disease treatment, research, and policy. In our extended allegory, the original gardener has retired (but is still voting), and a new gardener has taken over. By that time, a few pink-blossoming seeds have blown into the rich soil, taken root, and flourished (as well as anyone could in the shade of the towering red-blossomed plants.) Some bees have pollinated pink blossoms with red pollen and red blossoms with pink pollen. As a result, new plants are taking on every shade between the original bubblegum pink and scarlet red. Now, the new gardener knows the history of the flower boxes and sees the differences in soil between them but doesn't feel like they should be held responsible for the sins of their predecessor, so they just add a layer of fertile soil to each flower box.

One day a young botanist happens by and notices how, on average, the red-blossoming plants are flourishing compared to the scrawny pink-blossoming plants. They suspect the disparity in growth is related to blossom color. They see the blossoms range from bubblegum pink to scarlet red and everything in between. They notice plant heights vary from weak and short to tall and healthy. The botanist associates scrawniness with pink blossoms, reasoning that because blossom color is inherited, so must be the ability to grow. And if they were being fully honest, they weren't even sure the pink-blossoming plants have an ancestor in common with the red ones. Like, sure, the pink-blossoming plants are technically plants, just not from the same genetic stuff that yielded the red-blossoming plants.

The new gardener suspects the same, and while they didn't have the money or will to change out the original poor rocky soil, they are able to grant generous funding to the botanist to isolate the specific genes that prevent the pink flowers from growing. The botanist begins their analysis by extracting and sequencing the DNA of the red and pink plants. The genomes are 99.9% identical, so the botanist determines they must share the same origin, but is confident that the 0.1% difference will explain the scrawniness.

By now, in the larger society, referring to plant blossoms solely by their color—especially given the varying blossom shades—has come to be thought of as crude and unscientific, so the botanist decides it would be more precise to categorize the plants by what percentage of their DNA corresponds to their color. On average, the higher the percentage of pink DNA, the scrawnier the plant, so the botanist concludes that pink DNA is a risk factor for scrawniness. The new gardener, intrigued by these findings, provides even more funding to allow the botanist to continue this work, to the exclusion of work examining the original flower box environments and conditions. Eventually, the botanist discovers a genetic variant that appears to be associated with growth in the red plants and a slightly different variant in the pink plants. They recommend investigations to determine how the variant contributes to growth and gene manipulation experiments to target and modify the pink mutation.

In our extended allegory, the new gardener represents how opinions and ideologies are being passed down through generations without question and then reinforced by skewed funding for genetics research. This inherited dogma follows on the heels of the original gardener, who created the hierarchy based on blossom color, just as colonization historically rooted in White supremacy created political hierarchies based upon race and skin color. These political hierarchies are still felt today because they shaped institutions such as the prison and educational systems and housing and job markets that perpetuate systems of inequity—all of which affect health. The insufficient research on developing measures to assess structural and institutional levels of racism and the inadequate funding dedicated to research focused on structural racism are reflective of the bias inherent in biomedical research.

The botanist is akin to researchers focusing on identifying race-specific disease-causing alleles (or gene variants), even though in 2000 the Human Genome Project announced there was no biological basis for race because human DNA was 99.9% identical. They still think their hunt is legitimate because 0.1% is still like a million genetic combinations and because some disorders are caused by a change in one gene, like sickle cell disease and Tay-Sachs disease that predominate in African and Ashkenazi Jewish populations, without acknowledging the regional geographic origin of both diseases—things like deserts, mountains, oceans, or religions keep people from making babies with other groups of people for hundreds of generations. That racial patterns in complex diseases like hypertension and cancer arise through multiple gene interactions with surrounding conditions, such as nutrition, toxic environmental exposures, and psychosocial stress, usually goes unacknowledged as well.

The botanist begins with an attempt to show that the plants are not even of the same progenitor—similarly, scientists and physicians during the 18th and 19th centuries attempted to prove races were biologically distinct subspecies and not merely sociopolitical inventions. Next, they made a conscious, a priori decision to stratify the analysis by color, based on their assumption that blossom color is genetically linked to growth. Although blossom color is inherited, there was no evidence that blossom color was genetically linked to growth independent of soil conditions. In much the same way, modern geneticists often stratify by socially assigned race at the start of genome-wide association studies to search for disease-causing alleles—researchers reason that because the phenotypic characteristics used to define race are inherited and worse outcomes appear in specific racial categories, race must be a reasonable proxy for disease-causing alleles. But as depicted in this allegory, no evidence suggests that alleles encoding characteristics such as skin color and hair texture also encode specific disease phenotypes. In fact, no genetic causation can be attributed to any phenotypic presentation unless the populations in question have shared the same environment—a situation made impossible by the disparate soil environments for the plants in this allegory and by structural racism for human populations.

The botanist's decision to rename the blossoms not on the basis of color but rather according to the percentages of pink or red DNA resembles how modern researchers have rebranded language from "race" to "ancestry." Ancestry is a more refined and specific alternative to race, many researchers claim, because ancestry estimates are inferred from objective informative markers in the genome, rather than by self-report. These markers are derived, however, from living reference populations being treated as "ancestors" and often defined by whole continents—for instance, Africa and Europe—which historically have served as delineations for racial categorizations. Therefore, defining percentages of African ancestry and European ancestry cannot be independent of the phenotypic presentations of those continental regions, especially since the phenotypic presentations reflect decisions that result in structural, mediated, and internalized racism. Said another way, one cannot assume that a higher proportion of African ancestry is evidence of a genomic contribution to a complex disease, since these associations are confounded by the experiences of racism and anti-Blackness that are also associated with African ancestry and darker skin color.

Returning to our allegory, once the botanist finds the growth gene variant, they attribute it to differing ancestries and go down a path of gene therapy rather than considering that the plants' interactions with the environment can alter gene expression and activity. In short, this example represents the way in which researchers suggest ancestry can serve as a proxy for disease-causing alleles and capture the contribution of structural racism to health outcomes, but without testing any specific measures of structural racism. This shortcut perpetuates a misguided assumption that every person within a population experiences the same aspects of racism to the same degree—without consideration of individual exposure to social determinants of health driven by racism in its various forms, such as whether or how long an individual has lived in a neighborhood where they are disproportionately exposed to pollution, or whether or how long an individual is exposed to personally mediated racism and their physiological response to it.

Now imagine what would have happened had the botanist thought to approach the research by investigating how the flower boxes differed. From there, they would have discovered the soil as the true source of the growth disparity. With further examination, the botanist would find proximity to poor soil directly and inversely correlates with plant growth, which would have led to the solution that would resolve the disparity: replacing the poor soil and subpar environment with fertile soil and creating the conditions for the pink-blossoming plants that allowed the red-blossoming plants to flourish in the first place.

What if researchers today did the same and focused their attention on resolving the structures of racism that created our disparities, instead of continuing a fruitless quest to find a genetic culprit? Even now, most medical journals won't even publish the word racism. In a 2021 *Health Affairs* article, "Medicine's Privileged Gatekeepers: Producing Harmful Ignorance About Racism and Health," Krieger and colleagues describe their analysis of articles published in leading medical journals—*New England Journal of Medicine, The Lancet, Journal of the American Medical Association,* and *British Medical Journal*—between January 1, 1990, and December 31, 2020. The *New England Journal of Medicine* was the worst. Of 43,378 articles published, only 109 included the word "racism" anywhere in the text, and just 4 of those were empirical research studies—and then only as a passing mention in the discussion section as a possible explanation for observed patterns or part of the infamous "more research is needed" concluding statements.

I don't know what it will take for Medicine to ask itself what the utility of Black-White comparisons is. Or at what point will Medicine acknowledge why the race-based comparisons were ever made at all? Getting there will require that the biomedical sciences abandon the notion of "race" and its derivations and recognize that these terms are nothing more than products of White supremacist ideology.

But whenever there is a conversation about the need to abolish race-based Medicine, the legacy of racism rears its ugly head. Someone once recounted a story of a Black man who lay dying of sepsis in the ICU after the team had tried everything. The patient was being treated with the appropriate antibiotics and all the vasopressors, but still the blood pressure refused to rise. When the patient survived, it was argued that because of race-based medicine, this patient's life was saved. All because of methylene blue.

For patients in septic shock, methylene blue can be a lifesaver. It can increase blood pressure, reduce the time needed on other vasopressors, decrease the time spent in the ICU, and lessen time on mechanical ventilation. But if you have G6PD enzyme deficiency, methylene blue can kill you.

Now, I don't know if this patient left the hospital with a good portion of his limbs, organs, and brain cells intact, but at least he survived the team's loud and wrong race-based medicine. They got it exactly backward; they believed methylene blue was safe to try *because* the patient was Black. See, roughly 2% of the general population has this condition, which, like sickle cell disease, evolved from humanity's need to survive malaria. Because G6PD deficiency is X-linked and malaria is endemic to sub-Saharan Africa and the Mediterranean, roughly 1 in 10 African American men will have G6PD deficiency. So in truth, the team's race-based rationale put the patient in more harm's way. Everyone was just fortunate they were wrong. But even if they had been right, using race as a surrogate for genetic predisposition is ridiculous. Because instead of making assumptions and gambling with someone's life, they could have just tested for the disease.

PART II
RACE DISREGARDED

CHAPTER 4

MELANIN AND LOCKS

With all the conversation about "Black kidneys," "Black lungs," and single-digit DNA patterns, one would think Medicine would not overlook the characteristics that *actually* distinguish most Black people from White people: skin color and hair texture. One would be wrong.

As a young child, I remember looking quizzically at the crayon labeled "flesh-colored" because it wasn't remotely the same color as my flesh. But I just kept it moving to the brown crayon to more accurately depict my portraits of self and family. It's not so simple in Medicine. Rashes can look drastically different on darker versus lighter skin shades, yet the textbooks and lectures have traditionally focused on fair skin.

The one exception is the depiction of the rashes and ulcers of sexually transmitted diseases. Here we get a plethora of Black penises. A Black penis with the classic chancre sore of syphilis. A Black penis with clusters of warts. A Black penis with a cluster of vesicles. Black penis, Black penis, Black PENIS! So many Black penises that one would think Black men, and only Black men, are out here fucking indiscriminately without condoms, which, of course, perpetuates the stereotype of Black promiscuity.

The result of centering fair skin in most other cases is that rashes are missed and diagnoses are delayed for people with darker skin. The classic example is the "bullseye" rash of tick-spread Lyme disease. What looks like a Target logo on fairer skin looks more like a purplish bump on darker skin, which explains why Black people experience brain and heart issues related to the late signs of the disease.

As I first told in my piece "California Dermatologists Offer Equitable Care to Dark-Skinned Patients" for the California Health Care Foundation (CHCF) blog, I experienced my first real-life lesson in how this disregard can harm patients as a resident physician.[1] I was summoned to the emergency room to evaluate a young Black man thought to have blood clots in both legs, clots that could dislodge, travel to the lungs, and cause death. The other doctors suspected deep vein thrombosis because both his lower legs were swollen. I was wary of the preliminary diagnosis because it would be unusual for an active young man to develop a clot, and even more unlikely for anyone to develop clots in both legs at once. Having been raised in a family whose skin colors ranged from black coffee to a cup with three creams, when I examined the patient, I could see what the White doctors could not. The patient's normal skin color was dark brown. Red, quarter-sized bumps tender to the touch dotted both shins. It was clear to me that it was erythema nodosum. Fluffy projections seen straddling his trachea on a chest x-ray—hilar adenopathy—reinforced my suspicions. This young man had sarcoidosis, a disease in which multiple tiny clumps of white blood cells and other tissue form primarily in the lungs but can also deposit in the skin, bones, nervous, and gastrointestinal systems. It is an entirely different diagnosis than blood clots—and would not respond to the powerful and potentially dangerous intravenous blood thinners indicated for deep vein thrombosis.

I believe this miss had to do with the common teaching that sarcoid is a disease of Black women. In *Hundreds of Interlaced Fingers*, I recounted the story of a renowned rheumatologist who, during a lunchtime lecture he hosted when I was in residency training, presented a case of a 40-something-year-old Black woman with a cough, shortness of breath, weight loss, and the same large tender bumps on shin and x-ray findings as the young Black man I described. The rheumatologist explained that the diagnosis in the case was delayed for years. It turned out, the 60-something-year-old White man was describing his own history but couldn't see past his own deeply held stereotypes.

Drs. Jenna Lester and Nada Elbuluk, two Black women dermatologists I interviewed for the CHCF article, shared stories of dangerous stereotypes, including instances where providers incorrectly assumed that Black people don't get skin cancers like melanoma. This assumption can lead to late or missed diagnoses of those cancers. The risk of melanoma for Black people is thought to be roughly 20 times lower than the risk for White people, but it is not zero. As a result, Black people tend to be diagnosed with skin cancer at more advanced stages, which results in worse outcomes. The survival rate five years after diagnosis is 90% for White patients with melanoma; for Black patients, it is 66%.[2]

Lester recounted the story of a Black patient whose primary care doctor misdiagnosed a melanoma skin growth as a keloid—a raised overgrowth of scar tissue that results from an excessive repair process at the site of a skin injury. While it is assumed keloids more commonly develop in darker-skinned people, clinicians must still consider other diagnoses. This misdiagnosis and mistreatment went on for months before a dermatologist was finally consulted, and at that point, it was too late to avert the patient's preventable death from skin cancer.

Of note, I had to change the CHCF version of this story, in which I wrote, "While keloids more commonly develop. . . ." Although keloids have been reported to develop around 15 times more frequently for darker-skinned people (more on that study forthcoming), that is not a high enough percentage or a good enough reason to diagnose and dismiss a patient without considering other possibilities.[3] This goes to show how ingrained these teachings are. We have already covered how racial assumptions can influence the findings in medical journals and academia, and we will explore more examples in this chapter. Even I, someone who was writing about anti-Black stereotypes, had failed to question the common teaching that it is "a fact" that keloids are more common in darker-pigmented skin.

Once, my red-headed, blue-eyed, fair-skinned friend Laura Plantinga told me about an experience her similarly blue-eyed and fair-skinned (but dirty-blonde-haired) sister had. "Must have one in the woodpile," an older surgeon, a White man, said when he saw the keloids that formed around an abdominal surgical scar from her teenage years. In his mind, the only way to explain such an unexpected finding was to assume that somewhere in the family tree was some African ancestry.

Dr. Andrea T. Deyrup, a pathology course director for Duke University School of Medicine, takes on this topic as part of her YouTube series "Pathology Central: Race in Medicine."[4] In this series, she delves into the literature under-pinning each assertion of a race-based disparity mentioned in the textbook *Robbins Basic Pathology 10th Edition*.[5] When met with the textbook's statement "Certain individuals seem to be predisposed to keloid formation, particularly those of African descent," Deyrup acknowledges that she assumed that a "deep dive" could be accomplished by sticking one's big toe into a shallow pond. But then she took a step and found herself engulfed in a sea of "misinformation, lies, poor study design, and structural racism."

For this series, she collaborated with Dr. Joseph Graves Jr., an evolutionary biology professor at North Carolina A&T State University, the country's largest historically Black university. (As a North Carolina native, I'm embarrassed I didn't know this about North Carolina A&T State University until she said it. I'll say more about why later.) The deep dive starts with two sentences from a paper entitled "Abnormal Wound Healing: Keloids" published by Robles and Berg in *Clinics in Dermatology* in 2007: "Overall, the risk of developing keloids is approximately 15 times higher in dark-skinned individuals compared with whites. The incidence of keloids in blacks and Hispanics varies from 4.5% to 16%, with higher incidences during puberty and pregnancy."[6]

Deyrup didn't have to do much to debunk the "15 times" assertion as pure misinformation. Robles and Berg cited a 2001 paper from Brissett and Sherris, who cited a 1969 paper by Alhady and Sivanantharajah in which they examined 175 cases of keloids in various races and found that "fair-skinned Chinese appear to be slightly more prone to keloids than the dark-skinned Indians and Malays."[7]

She did the math and found the ratio of keloids to be two to three times more common among dark-skinned people compared to fair-skinned people. With that finding, it appears Brissett and Sherris couldn't do simple math or get the ratio direction right. Yet their "15 times" remains in the literature. Alhady and Sivanantharajah go on to state that keloids "are commonest amongst Negroes, the reported Negro:white ratio varying from 2:1 to 14:1," citing a 1953 paper by Kitlowski, which doesn't mention a prevalence at all, and a 1954 paper by Allan and Keen, which reported on a study of a predominantly African (Bantu) population where fewer fair-skinned people were present for comparison.[8]

Of note, the Robles and Berg paper is what the editor of UpToDate quoted in response to Deyrup's 2021 request that they omit the phrase "of African descent." In addition to cosigning the Brissett and Sherris "15 times" misinformation, the Robles and Berg paper also references a 2002 paper by Aköz and colleagues about treating earlobe keloids in Turkey. Aköz and colleagues, in turn, cite three other papers to justify the claim that "the incidence of keloids in blacks and Hispanics varies from 4.5% to 16%."[9] The first citation was a 1961 paper by Cosman and colleagues about patients in their New York clinic who had keloids.[10] Seventy-four percent of their patients were "Negro" and three times as many of them had keloids compared to their White patients.[11] They go on to cite two 1931 non-peer-reviewed reports from a dermatologic meeting where one group reported 4.5% and 13.3% of Swiss schoolchildren and adults, respectively, had keloids and another reported that 16% of Congolese mine workers had keloids.[12]

Deyrup points out that the low prevalence among schoolchildren speaks to the fact that keloids are a product of scars, so getting them is more likely to accrue with living through injuries, surgeries, tattoos, and piercings. She further argues that there is little clinical difference between 13.3% and 16%, at least not enough to make sure generations of medical students have this notion hardwired into their memory.

By this point, one may be asking, "Why bother stipulating that keloids are more common in darker-skinned people?" Because of the effects of anti-Blackness.

Although keloids are benign and clinically non-consequential, they can be disfiguring. The assumption they would be more common in the "deeply pigmented, swarthy, oily skin" of the Negro as opposed to the "light, thin, dry skin" of Whites is a product of racist assumptions.[13] But that's what Koonin, the author of the second paper cited by Aköz and colleagues, wrote in his 1964 paper (which he plagiarized from Kitlowski). If this all seems convoluted and circular, it's because it is. Misinformation, poor study design, lies, and structural racism usually are. Yet racism is so embedded in society that, as plastic surgeon Ivens C. Leflore pointed out in his 1980 publication "Misconceptions Regarding Elective Plastic Surgery in the Black Patient" in the *Journal of the National Medical Association*, Black people may be reluctant to get surgery due to fear about developing disfiguring keloids, when in truth one only need look at how past skin traumas healed, rather than the color of their skin, to know if they are prone to keloids.[14]

Lester and Elbuluk also point out that providers ignoring the distinguishing characteristics of Black people doesn't have to be fatal to have a significant impact on someone's life. For example, lacking awareness around grooming practices and preferences outside a White-centered norm can harm patients. They describe an encounter where doctors assumed that a Black woman with straight hair had used a chemical "relaxer" to straighten her hair, but she had only used heated appliances. They also recount a doctor recommending a Black woman use a corticosteroid shampoo several times a week to treat dandruff. When her condition hadn't improved a month later, the doctors were confused because they hadn't bothered to ask about her usual hair care routine. Often Black people, unlike people with naturally straight and more oil-producing hair, have a weekly or biweekly "wash day." While there is no overarching hair care routine for all Black people and some may wash their hair daily, the doctors did not ask about the patient's practices, because they were working off assumptions based on White people's, and likely their own, grooming practices. All they had to do was ask her. Providers' failure to adapt their treatment recommendations commonly results in patients leaving the exam room feeling unheard and unseen.

One such patient is Hilary Alexis.

I knew Hilary from a book club and admired how she confidently rocked a smooth dome, long before Congresswoman Ayanna Pressley made it look cool. But I learned it took her a while to get there.

She was in her forties when she noticed her hairline receding. She told her primary care doctor, a White man around her age who was experiencing male-pattern baldness himself. He didn't think Alexis's hair loss was cause for concern. He sent her to the lab to check her B vitamins and thyroid function. When those results came back within normal limits, she said, the doctor shrugged. In subsequent visits, she repeatedly raised the issue of her hair loss, and he said, "I don't know," and never even suggested a dermatology referral.

"I don't think it would have been dismissed by a Black doctor," she said.

Years later, she consulted two dermatologists on her own. By then, however, her undiagnosed condition had passed the point of no return, and she was essentially doing a comb-over with artificial two-strand braids (twists) to cover her retreating hairline.

"I had a full-on Barnum and Bailey clown hairline," she said. "The fake twists were just another form of clownishness." She finally shaved her head for the first time in 2016.

Medicine's disregard for non-White skin color has even seeped into the equipment. Medicine did not consider skin color when it would truly matter: testing the accuracy of pulse oximeters. The pulse oximeter, or pulse ox, invented in the 1970s, is an electronic device that painlessly measures the saturation of oxygen carried in one's red blood cells in seconds. The device is clipped onto a part of the body, usually the fingertip, but it could be the nose, ears, or toes. It emits a light on one side of the body part, and a sensor on the other side measures the amount of light not absorbed by the fingernail, skin, tissue, and blood to calculate the oxygen saturation. A normal oxygen saturation is 95% and above. Less than 90% indicates a need for medical attention.

It makes sense that factors like scar tissue and skin pigment would affect readings. Nevertheless, the pulse ox was tested in predominantly fair-skinned populations. In a *New England Journal of Medicine* letter to the editor published on

December 16, 2020, Sjoding and colleagues reported that in two large cohorts, pulse oximetry read oxygen saturation of 92% to 96% when the directly measured blood oxygen saturation was less than 88% nearly three times more often in Black patients than in White patients.[15] During my medical training, it was common knowledge that fingernail polish would give an inaccurate reading, but the accuracy of readings was never questioned for darker-skinned patients.

I wasn't aware of pulse ox overestimating oxygen saturation in Black people when my piece "The Health Care System Has the Black Community in a Choke Hold" was published by the California Health Care Foundation blog in 2020.[16] In it I share a story told by Dr. Sheila Young, a physician-scientist and director of the free COVID-19 testing site on the campus of Charles R. Drew University of Medicine and Science in South Los Angeles, about a Black woman with shortness of breath. It was the woman's third trip to the emergency department, and she was starting to panic. She knew the COVID-19 death toll was climbing and that it was far worse for Black people than White people, and yet the doctors told her to go home again. But this time she pleaded, "If you all don't admit me to the hospital, I'm going to die. I can't breathe."

"'I can't breathe.' This is a sentiment we've heard before," Young said.

When New York City police took Eric Garner into custody for selling loose cigarettes in 2014, we heard him say "I can't breathe" before he died in a police officer's choke hold. On May 25, after Minneapolis police accused George Floyd of passing a counterfeit $20 bill, we heard him say "I can't breathe" as he begged Derek Chauvin, the officer kneeling on his neck, to release him. Chauvin, his hands resting in his pockets as if he were strolling through the park, didn't budge until Floyd was dead.

And during the pandemic, we increasingly heard it from Black people at the mercy of the American health care system. A system that is literally supposed to help those who can't breathe is figuratively applying a choke hold to Black people by sending them home to die when they say "I can't breathe."

Gary Fowler, a 56-year-old Black man, was denied COVID-19 testing and hospital admission by three Detroit emergency rooms where he complained of difficulty breathing. Deshaun Taylor, a 23-year-old Black man, was sent home twice from a Chicago hospital, even after testing positive. Reginald Relf, a 50-year-old Black man, was turned away from an urgent care clinic in suburban Chicago without being tested despite his labored breathing, fever, and cough. Kimora Lynum, a 9-year-old Black girl with a fever of 103 degrees, was sent home from a Florida academic medical center without being tested. They all died soon after.

From 2019 to 2020, the Black population had the second-largest increase in deaths, next to the American Indian and Alaskan Native populations.[17] In February 2021, the Food and Drug Administration issued an alert on the limitations of pulse oximeters.[18] I wonder how often pulse ox readings were used to justify clinicians' decisions to sentence Black people to death prior to an alert to something known for decades.

CHAPTER 5

BLACK VOICES UNHEARD

In my first year at Duke Medical School, I was among five medical students led by two faculty members who watched silently as a sixth student practiced interviewing a young Black man playing the role of a patient with sickle cell disease. Our "patient" was a person who had just moved to the area and was in pain and need of medicine to relieve it. These were the days before electronic medical records, so confirming a medical history took days. The patient was hurting now. After a lot of back and forth between the patient and my White male peer, one of the faculty decided to call a time-out for discussion. My all-White peers and the faculty discussed concerns about the patient's increasing urgency around the need for opiates. I finally said, "Are we so hesitant to give him pain medicine because he is Black?"

A hush fell over the room.

Our patient's back was turned to us during the time-out, but I could sense he was glad somebody acknowledged the elephant in the room. And that's when the student interviewer said, "I don't see color." That was the first time I heard that cliché, but it wouldn't be the last.

Having lived a sheltered, nerd-child life in rural North Carolina until leaving for college, I didn't know enough about Medicine (or even the world) to confidently call bullshit in my medical school pretend patient experience. What I've learned since then is that while Medicine professes to be color-blind, what it repeatedly demonstrates is that it cannot *hear* people of color. When Black people speak, Medicine does not listen. Or refuses to believe what Black people say through the noise of their biases.

One of my most poignant examples of being unheard happened on May 16, 2019. I was set to present to the Medical Executive Committee at Zuckerberg San Francisco General Hospital (ZSFG). My PowerPoint presentation that read "The Case for a Standard Clinical Ethics Consultation Service" in the brand colors, navy and white, along with logos for both UCSF and ZSFG was cued up. As the committee's name implies, all the hospital bigwigs sat around the small conference room's standard rectangular table. I, co-chair of the Ethics Committee, had the floor for 10 minutes.

Apart from the brown print scarf I put over my hair and then twisted into a bun in the back, I don't remember what I wore that day. My makeup was natural and understated. The look was no-nonsense to match my tone. I've never been one of those people who could smile and talk about serious topics at the same time.

My first slide explained how the committee convened monthly or ad hoc whenever the hospital medical teams found themselves in a quandary, such as if a patient's family wanted to continue the intensive care the doctors deemed futile or incapable of producing a meaningful result. But most families found their loved one's beating heart and any brain activity extremely meaningful and worth the ventilator, maximum intravenous medicines, multiple tubes, and, occasionally, a constant dialysis machine—while they waited for their miracle. The committee existed to cosign and approve the hospital physicians' plans to run roughshod over the families' wishes and pull all the plugs while reassuring them that doing so was ethical and right. After hours' worth of meetings where I heard only the physicians' perspectives on the ethical principles of beneficence, non-maleficence, justice, and autonomy, I had become disillusioned and stopped going to meetings altogether. As the only Black person in regular attendance and the only Black doctor on the committee, I felt an obligation to attend. Somebody needed to mirror the mostly minoritized population the hospital served. So when I was invited to be co-chair, I decided to return to the committee and advocate for change from within.

I wanted us to do better. I wanted us to meet the standards of clinical ethics consultation per the American Society for Bioethics and Humanities.[1] I had a slide of what that looked like: us reviewing the health record, documenting in the medical record, and compiling firsthand perspectives from all involved. I had a slide where I shared examples of how talking to the patient and family made a tremendous difference. A slide that made the business case for an ethics consultation service—five fewer days in the ICU and clinical consensus means less money spent. Another slide detailing how a service was aligned with our "True North" goals. Still another slide about how division chiefs wanted a clear process, documentation in the medical record, and engagement of all involved in patient cases. Finally, a slide on potential grants that would fund such services—which I estimated to cost less than what I'd imagine the hospital spent on toilet paper—while we demonstrated cost savings that would justify making it part of the hospital's operating budget. I hoped the hospital leadership could be on board with that. I ended my presentation, thanked them for their time and attention, and excused myself.

While I did not expect to walk out of that room with a five-figure check, I didn't expect what I got. After the meeting, a top-ranking hospital executive approached me in the hallway to say, "What was *that*, Vanessa? You basically just called us all unethical!"

I looked around for the cameras. Surely, I was getting punked. Then I realized this top-ranking executive was serious, and all the audience had taken away from my presentation was hurt feelings. That day, I learned people interpret anything I say filtered through the biases, conscious or unconscious, they hold toward the Black-woman package I live in. That person apologized to me a few weeks later—but then asked for the same information I had presented to the committee, further demonstrating they hadn't heard an actual word I said. This example may be understood as having an indirect effect on patients; the examples of direct neglect are plentiful.

In Wanda Sykes's May 2019 Netflix special *Not Normal,* she jokes about how doctors diminish Black people's pain and reserve opioids for White pain. "I had a double mastectomy," she shares, "You know what they sent my Black ass home with? I-bu-fucking-profen." Her sentiments were confirmed just a few months later in the article "A 'Rare Case Where Racial Biases' Protected African-Americans" published in *The New York Times.* The article's authors speculate that the opioid overdose death rate among White people is twice that of Black people because doctors gave fewer opioid prescriptions to Black people. They theorize that because doctors believed Black people would be more likely to become addicted to the drugs, would be more likely to sell the drugs, and "had a higher pain threshold than white people because they were biologically different," they wrote them fewer opioid scripts.[2] While some have suggested this false belief resulted in a good, protective disparity, I'd bet these are the same people who never had to face unrelenting pain with i-bu-fucking-profen.

This is no laughing matter for patients like Aaron Lloyd, a real-life example of the actor-patient with sickle cell disease from medical school. Besides Aaron, there are more than 100,000 other Americans with the disease, the vast majority of whom are Black. But it's this "vast majority" that Medicine tends to focus on, so much so that sickle cell is commonly called a "Black" disease. In truth, it is a *geographical* disease that can affect anyone from any racial group. Nature created a slight variation in the gene that makes blood to protect against malaria, a potentially deadly disease caused by the Anopheles mosquito found in sub-Saharan Africa *and* South America, the Caribbean, Central America, Saudi Arabia, India, and Mediterranean countries. Children inherit this gene. Inheritance of one copy of the gene variant confers protection from malaria, while inheriting two copies (one from each parent) results in sickle cell disease. Typical red blood cells are round and move through the tiniest of blood vessels to deliver oxygen to all the parts of the body, but in sickle cell disease, these cells become distorted into hard sickle shapes. Sickle blood cells die early, causing constant anemia. These cells get stuck in blood vessels, causing strokes, infections, and many other life-shortening problems. Sickle cell disease also causes bouts of pain so bad the medical term for them is "pain crises."

Vaccinations, medications, and screenings given to newborns to check for sickle cell disease have drastically improved how long people live; in the 1970s, people with sickle cell disease lived less than 20 years on average. However, newborn screening has only been ubiquitous in the United States, Puerto Rico, and the Virgin Islands since 2006.

Born in 1967, Aaron wasn't diagnosed with sickle cell disease until he was five years old. He was sure he had pain crises before then, but at five, all his little limbs were so swollen and bruised that he was taken to the ER.

Still, Aaron considered himself lucky, lucky to get care in a specialty clinic alongside other children with sickle cell disease and other illnesses such as cystic fibrosis and leukemia. He read comic books designed for children with sickle cell disease and learned tips for avoiding pain crises. The proximity to other children's suffering and deaths gave him a broader perspective. It may have even helped him work through coming to terms with his illness, what he calls his "why me?" phase, a little sooner.

He felt particularly fortunate to have been under the care of just two hematologists throughout his treatment. Aaron saw a pediatric hematologist until he was 21. Now he sees an adult hematologist. Fortunate, because he saw his hematologists as "saviors" when the pain crises came. Only they could shield him from the ER doctors' and nurses' assumptions as he aged out from being a sick child to a Black man complaining of pain.

"It's like a 180 flip," he said comparing the change in care. "All the nurturing care given to the sick child ends at 18 and becomes very cold and clinical." In this instance, he was grateful for his baby face, as it likely bought him some time.

"Reputation is everything," Aaron said of being in the ER. One doesn't want to be labeled noncompliant in their medical record for fear the next stranger in the ER will read that and let it color their perception. Simply resisting what the doctor recommends can get one labeled as such. Even if you are a patient who knows what will and won't work based on consistent medical experiences and time spent in hospitals, you will not be believed. He recalls a time when he was given hydromorphone, commonly known as Dilaudid. The drug caused him to have strange compulsive behaviors such as stacking items and folding paper into smaller and smaller squares. After his concerns went unheard, rather than arguing with ER staff, his wife asked that he be transferred to the hospital where he usually received care.

Another time, he remembers begging an ER nurse to be sure to carefully swab the port at his left upper chest that facilitated blood draws and pain medication. It was his fourth port. The first three had to be removed after another nurse's sloppy technique resulted in infections. "Why, are you using it to shoot heroin?" the nurse replied.

Aaron had never used drugs, drank alcohol, or smoked because he knew each could lead to a pain crisis; on top of that, he wasn't even aware that people could use a port for injecting drugs. The remark hurt him deeply.

Every time he went to the ER, he felt he had to clear hurdles to prove himself worthy of care. He had to be his best self when he felt his worst. He knew that tears or crying out in pain would get one quickly labeled as drug-seeking. But stoicism would be misinterpreted by nurses as a sign that he wasn't truly in pain. The slights, assumptions, and accusations—on top of excruciating pain—often became overwhelming, which was why Aaron would only consider going to the ER when his prescribed dose of morphine pills was not enough to bring the pain down to a tolerable level.

This kind of performance—Aaron's careful dance of "appropriately" exhibiting pain while experiencing excruciating levels of it—is an echo of the 1840s "science" that claimed Black people don't feel pain in the first place, at least not as strongly as White people. It wasn't until a 1961 publication led by Dr. John Thomas, a renowned Black physician and researcher, that another explanation for the difference in Black vs. White responses to pain was introduced.[3] Thomas attributed differences in his findings from prior studies to others having misinterpreted more stoicism among Black patients compared to White patients as a lack of pain. He also explained that Black people may use different words to describe pain than White people. For example, some denied pain but reported "indigestion" or that they were "hurting" in the chest. He noted the 13–14% percent of Black patients described as having no pain were all either "unconscious or irrational" due to other complicating factors like severe heart failure or stroke. He postulated that the shortness of breath that came with the onset of heart failure may have taken precedence over previous pain if the patient was not questioned carefully.

Aaron's account of everyday life shows how pain is treated depending on one's race. One study published in the *Journal of the National Medical Association* in 2007 found that physicians across 12 primary care centers were twice as likely to underestimate pain in Black patients compared to all other races combined.[4] A review of the literature on the relationship between pain and race published by the American Medical Association in 2013 cited studies in which despite higher pain scores than White patients, Black and Latinx patients were less likely to receive any pain medication, received lower doses of pain medication, and were more likely to wait longer for pain medication in the ER.[5]

Perhaps more surprising is that the teaching about pain differences by race continues. In 2012, *Pain Medicine* published a systematic literature review and analysis of 26 studies using experimental pain stimuli to test pain sensitivity across various racial groups. All studies were published from 1944 to 2011.[6] At the time of this writing, the review article was still cited in the "Cultural Aspects of Palliative Care: Issues Related to Pain, Suffering, and Distress" section of UpToDate, the popular, evidence-based clinical resource for health care providers since 1992, demonstrating how unethical research gets passed on as truth to providers who are tasked with taking care of patients like Aaron.

But these differences in treatment can't be dismissed as assumptions about "Black genes." As I wrote in my piece "Researchers Seek Reproductive Justice for Black Women" published by the California Health Care Foundation blog in 2020, this belief is a symptom of Medicine's racism.[7]

Consider that Black mothers die in hospitals at nearly four times the rate of White mothers. This disgraceful disparity has persisted for decades despite state and national quality improvement initiatives, clinical safety innovations, and technological advances.[8] It persists regardless of patient income, insurance, education, comorbid conditions, or prenatal care.

Anthropologist Dr. Dána-Ain Davis explains in her book *Reproductive Injustice: Racism, Pregnancy, and Premature Birth* that "obstetric racism" takes many forms.[9] Seven to be exact, which can be applied across Medicine.

There is the "medical abuse" form of obstetric racism dating back to 19th-century physician J. Marion Sims, whose experimentation on enslaved Black women without anesthesia earned him the moniker "the father of modern gynecology." The "diagnostic lapses" form arises from de-emphasizing or ignoring patients' symptoms, as seen in the story of Kira Johnson, who bled to death after what was supposed to be a routine cesarean section. Her Black husband, Charles, noticed blood in her bladder catheter and brought it to doctors' and nurses' attention, but a CT scan didn't happen for another seven hours. That Charles hesitated to speak up forcefully in his advocacy for her out of fear the police would be called is an example of the "ceremonies of degradation" form of racism.

We learned that even celebrities aren't safe when Serena Williams exhibited the "racial reconnaissance" and "neglect, dismissiveness, or disrespect" forms after giving birth to her first child. Davis defines this form as Black women going to extreme efforts to avoid or mitigate racist encounters, including being hyper-vigilant about procedures and finding providers. Williams describes in her 2022 *Elle* magazine article, "How Serena Williams Saved Her Own Life," how the nurse tried to dismiss her insistence on getting a CT scan to diagnose clots in her lungs and the blood thinning medication to treat them, even though she had a history of lung clots seven years prior: "I think all this medicine is making you talk crazy," and telling her she just needed to go rest.[10]

Hell, not even doctors are safe. I experienced obstetric racism in the form of "coercion," when an ER provider admonished me, "You need to think about what's right for your baby!" when I refused the blood tests and an ambulance transfer to another hospital she recommended because I explained to her, my "practice" Braxton-Hicks contractions (which felt very real at the time) had already subsided. I did not want to stress my body out with tests and transfers when I knew I was fine. This type of intimidation when it comes to medical decisions, as well as medical professionals performing procedures without consent, is coercion.

And lest we forget Dr. Susan Moore, the family medicine physician who took to social media to broadcast how she exemplified the "intentionally causing pain" form of racism when a White doctor failed to manage her pain appropriately. "I put forth and I maintain if I was White," she says in her video, "I wouldn't have to go through that."[11] She felt she was treated like a drug addict. While an external investigation did not conclude her treatment, or lack of treatment, at Indiana University Health North contributed to her death just two weeks later, it did find that the doctor who treated Dr. Moore suffered from a "lack of cultural competence."

I wonder if the physician in Moore's case ever accepted the investigation's conclusion. Examples throughout Medicine suggest he likely did not. Unfortunately, the news is consistently littered with reports of physicians denying their own, as well as the medical field's, bias against the Black community.

On February 24, 2021, Medicine went even further and twisted their lips into saying, "No physician is racist, so how can there be structural racism in medicine?" These were words tweeted and repeated in a *JAMA Clinical Reviews* podcast by Dr. Edward Livingston, an associate editor of *Journal of the American Medical Association* (*JAMA*), the largest and oldest medical journal of the largest and oldest medical association in the US.[12] The tweet was intended to be clickbait to lure people to the 15-minute podcast where he and Dr. Mitch Katz, president and CEO of New York City Health and Hospitals—two White men—discussed "structural racism for skeptics."

Livingston started the podcast by admitting he didn't understand the concept of structural racism, because in his mind, racism—which he defined as the use of race to make decisions about what people can or can't do or somehow influence their possibilities—was made "patently illegal" with the passage of civil rights legislation in the 1960s. Therefore, given that racism is "illegal," he questioned how it could be so embedded in our society that it could be considered structural. Furthermore, he took offense to the term "racism" because he was raised not to see color.

In her book *PC, M.D.: How Political Correctness Is Corrupting Medicine* published in 2000, Dr. Sally Satel, psychiatrist, Yale lecturer, and scholar at the

American Enterprise Institute, a conservative think tank, argued that racial disparities in health care are often overblown and attributed to physician racism.[13] She claimed that focusing on systemic issues and socioeconomic factors, rather than accusing physicians of racism, was more productive.

In 2018, in a debate over racial disparities in care as part of the American Medical Association House of Delegates Resolution, Dr. James Madara, CEO of the organization, argued that "physicians, by the very nature of their work, cannot be racists."

In 2016, in response to concerns over health outcomes among Black children, Dr. Benard Dreyer, president of the American Academy of Pediatrics, said in an interview that "physicians are in the business of healing, not harm, so it's hard to imagine that they could hold racist views." Critics noted this overlooked implicit bias and its impact on pediatric care.

During a 2015 discussion on racial disparities in organ transplants, Dr. Anthony Monaco, former chair of the Organ Transplant Association, claimed that "physicians cannot be racist because the criteria for organ transplants are strictly medical."

During a medical school panel discussing implicit bias in clinical practice in 2014, Dr. Robert Weiss, a professor of medicine, argued that "physicians are trained in evidence-based medicine and cannot afford to be racist." This claim was contested by students and faculty who pointed to studies demonstrating racial disparities in patient treatment.

In 2021, during a public discussion on racial disparities in maternal mortality, Dr. William Schaffner, an infectious disease expert at Vanderbilt University, said, "It's hard to reconcile the idea that physicians could be racist when they're trying to save lives." His statement was criticized for disregarding the impact of racial bias on Black maternal health.

I could go on. Each of these examples highlights the dichotomy between the assertion that physicians are inherently neutral and the vast and ever-growing body of evidence showing that racial bias impacts health care outcomes beyond systemic issues. All these examples remind me of a line from the 2018 film *The Hate U Give*. In response to her White boyfriend's attempt to comfort her by saying he doesn't see her color, 18-year-old protagonist Starr cries, "If you can't see my color, you can't see me."

The same holds for Medicine. If Medicine can't hear a Black patient through their subconscious, and often overt, assumptions about the entire Black community or can't even acknowledge its role in the disparities plaguing Black people, how can Medicine properly take care of Black people?

CHAPTER 6

DIVERSITY AND THE SOCIAL DETERMINANTS OF SUCCESS

I come from a place where distances are measured by sweet potato fields, not neighborhood blocks. One could drive miles before reaching a stoplight. My high school was the kind of school where the SATs were just a day of coloring in bubbles with sharp number 2 pencils, and College Day featured technical schools, not Ivy League universities. Most of my classmates planned to get married right after graduation and stay in town. Many would end up working at the tire factory, and some would join the army.

The thought of becoming a doctor never occurred to me until my brother suggested I could. I hardly knew him because he was 16 years old when I was born and soon headed to the army. I didn't come from doctors, didn't know any doctors, and rarely saw a doctor. My family believed there was no need to see one when Robitussin, calamine lotion, and Vick's VapoRub cured all that ailed.

As a result, I may have been the worst medical student ever. I simply didn't get that it was all a game. A game I didn't know the rules to or have the playbook for. I liken it to when my son returned to football his senior year in high school after realizing shooting free throws like Shaquille O'Neal at *only* six-foot-three wasn't going to win him the Division 1 athletic scholarship he coveted. He had not played football since he was in sixth grade. The coach put him at the defensive end with the instruction, "Go knock down the quarterback." He was naturally good at it. He got 15 sacks that season and was named first-team best defensive player in the conference. But had he gotten the playbook earlier, he could have combined his natural talent with knowledge. That Division 1 football scholarship would have likely come easier and, with strategy, he may have been able to help his team win more games.

In Medicine, this playbook comes in the form of a "hidden curriculum," a set of implicit and unspoken rules, nuances, and knowledge one needs to know in order to be successful in medical training. The kinds of things children of doctors, lawyers, and professors get from direct conversation, osmosis, and internships gained through nepotism. The kinds of things Black people can lack access to, as ensured by a history of exclusion and oppression.

I call these the social determinants of success. Things that make it easier to get into and complete medical training. I planned to write an op-ed on the topic but could find no published data to back up my position. The closest was from the Association of American Medical Colleges but was limited to race and gender. So I sought to collect it myself as part of a larger study examining disciplinary experiences of resident physicians.

With the help of generous funding from the California Health Care Foundation and the Commonwealth Fund, this Institutional Review Board–approved study found that 19% of the 1,755 residents who completed the study survey were the first in their family to go to college, but 31% of Black residents were their family firsts. Sixty-one percent of participants reported they were the first in their family to earn any doctoral degree, but 76% of Black residents were their family firsts.[1] This legacy was created when Medicine established its first US medical school in 1765 but wouldn't admit and graduate a Black man, Dr. James McCune Smith, until 1847. They graduated their first White woman in 1849, but no Black woman until Dr. Rebecca Lee Crumpler in 1864.

Not surprisingly, poverty was overrepresented among Hispanic/Latinx and Black residents. While 22% of all participants reported growing up in a household of less than $50,000 annual income, 38% of Black residents grew up poor.

Just as people need certain conditions in their physical environments, socioeconomic standing, clinical health care, and their behaviors to be healthy—the social determinants of health—medical trainees need a certain set of conditions to succeed and thrive: the social determinants of success.

I remember performing poorly on microbiology exams until my classmate at the microscope to my right schooled me. Her name was Frances Eizember. She was a thin Asian woman with round glasses and curly hair. Frances had a career as an engineer before deciding to become a doctor. She explained that it didn't matter what you *actually* saw under the microscope. All that mattered was that you remembered what you were *supposed* to see. Memorize what you're supposed to see and write that down, she told me. She had scored a 98% on the last exam. I don't remember my score, but by the way I recall inhaling with stretched eyes tells me I hadn't come close. Luckily, I had the good sense to take her advice and become friends.

But I wasn't any better on the wards. On my first clinical rotation in pediatrics, I spent my time outside of rounds feeding and rocking the poor hospitalized babies. I thought that was how you showed you wanted to be a caring doctor. Meanwhile, my peers spent their downtime in the library. I performed so poorly on the end-of-service exam that the chief of pediatrics called me into his office to discuss it. I didn't know I was supposed to know you shouldn't give honey to babies in their first year. That kind of information didn't come from lectures or experience in the clinic setting. You were just supposed to know you had to go to the library and what book to read when you got there.

I didn't even get it during my fellowship. I fell into nephrology on a social justice mission to eliminate racial disparities in access to kidney transplants, not because of a fascination with electrolyte disorders and rare kidney diseases like my peers. And to make matters worse, I started my fellowship with a research year while my peers delved into clinical rotations. So when I finally hit clinical rotations, my attending physicians expected me to behave like a senior fellow. I was on the steep part of the learning curve. I didn't realize I was being tested during case presentations. I thought we were all chatting about an interesting case. I felt like I was in the way, just slowing down the work of my attendings, instead of providing the cheap labor they depended on to get their work done.

It is a wonder I survived. Yet I am an excellent doctor (if I do say so myself). I passed all my board examinations, including the internal medicine and nephrology boards on my first try. More meaningfully, my patients tell me how I make them feel heard, how thorough I am, and how effective my treatment plans are.

According to Dr. Norman Wang, cardiologist and coauthor of a white paper entitled "Diversity, Inclusion, and Equity: Evolution of Race and Ethnicity Consideration for the Cardiology Workforce in the United States of America from 1969 to 2019," I shouldn't have even been admitted to medical school.[2] His article was published in the *Journal of the American Heart Association* in March 2020. Apparently it took a few months for folks to catch up on their reading, because it wasn't until August that Twitter exploded in outrage, sadness, and disgust. The article was officially retracted soon thereafter.[3] The American Heart Association "became aware of serious concerns after publication. The author's institution, the University of Pittsburgh Medical Center (UPMC), has notified the Editor-in-Chief that the article contains many misconceptions and misquotes and that together those inaccuracies, misstatements, and selective misreading of source materials strip the paper of its scientific validity."[4]

Like every other troll that crawls out of the depths of social media any time the need for diversity in Medicine is mentioned, Wang argued that affirmative action policies result in admitting unqualified applicants and whipped out all the studies showing how MCAT scores vary by race. He specifically pointed out that White and Asian students with higher MCAT scores are less likely to be accepted into medical school than Black students with higher MCAT scores.

I don't even remember what my MCAT score was. All I know was that I took it once, because it was expensive. However, I was able to afford a prep course with my work-study earnings. Data from the Association of American Medical Colleges says that 39% of people who took the MCAT between 2020 and 2022 were re-testers (they had the money to take the MCAT multiple times) and many could afford private tutoring.[5]

But then, who cares? Not one patient has ever asked about my MCAT score. According to the Association of American Medical Colleges, MCAT scores predict how well someone will do in the first year of medical school. Nothing else. So instead of using the MCAT to determine if Black students are not good enough to be doctors, what if—and hear me out—we used the MCAT to identify which students might need extra support and gave them that support? As I wrote in my 2020 *New England Journal of Medicine* Points of View piece "Diversity, Equity, and Inclusion That Matter," Medicine should seriously consider what hardships candidates have endured to reach the same place as privileged candidates in order to create the workforce that can best understand and meet the needs of communities disproportionately affected by chronic illnesses.[6] These candidates may not fit all the criteria, because those criteria favor people who've always been highly favored. Just as test scores are biased toward those who can afford prep courses and repeat testing, letters of recommendation by those in positions of authority are often affected by racial bias. At some point, Medicine must decide to produce doctors who mirror the patient population, because cultural concordance improves patient outcomes.

As I wrote in "CMS Must Act to Ensure a Diverse Physician Workforce" for *Healthcare Business Today* in 2023, chronic disease and mortality are significantly higher among young adult Black Americans than among the US population.[7] According to the National Center for Health Statistics, Black Americans' life expectancy in 2020 was nearly 6 years shorter than non-Latinx White Americans.[8] Black American infants have a death rate of 10.8 deaths per 1,000 live births—almost twice the national average. But Black infant mortality is cut by half when they have Black doctors. The gap between Black and White men in cardiovascular mortality drops by 19% when Black men see a Black doctor. In counties with even one Black doctor, whether or not Black patients see those doctors, Black populations saw lower mortality from all causes and had lower disparities in mortality rates between Black and White residents. Having enough Black doctors saves lives. Yet Black physicians have made up only 4% of the physician workforce for decades.

Sadly, the likelihood of climbing the success ladder doesn't end just because medical training ends. At least within academia. Before I left UCSF, I was asked to serve on a search committee for a new chief of nephrology at the affiliated San Francisco Veterans Administration Medical Center. I don't remember if I was the only woman on the committee, but I was the only Black person there for sure. So while I check off *two* of the required diversity boxes for such searches, my voice was certainly never going to change the committee's recommendation for hire. I listened to them criticize a Black candidate for not having enough research publications, leadership positions, or grants while ignoring the fact that such accolades often come through mentorship and sponsorship, and ignoring how much time it took for this candidate to transform a residency program serving a mainly Black city from 1% Black to 20% Black in just five years. A CV thick with citations regardless of impact was considered much more valuable than recruiting a culturally concordant workforce. I referred to "CV thickness" in the same *New England Journal* article.[9]

In response to my point of view, there was this:

Jul 26, 2020

maintaining excellence

You ask for open dialogue.

My wife is Asian and immigrated at 5. Growing up poor in a rural, White town she experienced significant racism. A teacher even once lowered her sister's grade "because she didn't want an Asian graduating as valedictorian" (she, and all of her siblings did anyhow). Historically, "Chinese coolie" were treated as bad as Black slaves. Not only have Asian Americans suffered racism, but they also do not have the "400-year advantage" of which you speak. In fact, the MCAT, USMLE, etc. are probably more favorable toward Blacks than Asians since English is a second language for many of them.

And yet, Asians make up 17% of physicians while representing only 5.6% of the US population.

"Non-prototypical candidates with thinner CV's" sounds like a euphemism for "not as qualified." As a surgeon who treats patients, and as someone who has been on the receiving end of health care, I value thick CV's—irrespective of race or color. I understand that individual groups may face significant challenges, but rather than asking for lower standards, Asian Americans are instead quietly demonstrating that earning respect through rigorous hard work is a better policy.

Ahh, the old model-minority myth. White supremacy never tires of it. And what's up with trolls' obsession with the MCAT?

PART III
RACE DENIED

CHAPTER 7

HOW CAN MEDICINE BE RACIST

Despite all the blatant examples of how Medicine was at the forefront of race "science," the institution vehemently denies having anything in common with the dark beginnings of American society. Yet remnants of that legacy linger today. Medicine convinces themselves they are different by telling themselves, "I'm a good person/I became a doctor to help people, so how can I possibly be capable of such harm?" To them, Medicine is nothing like those cross-burning, mob-lynching, racial slur yellers. So how could Medicine be racist?

Never mind all the Black folks dying younger and at higher rates than everyone else. Medicine attributes all of that to forces outside itself. Those forces are just like all those "unmeasured genetic factors" Medicine's been searching for since the invention of Whiteness.

It took an act of Congress to get Medicine to face the reality that racial disparities do exist—even after access to care, patient preference, and appropriateness of intervention are taken off the table as the only reasons why. In 1999, Congress asked the Institute of Medicine to conduct a study assessing the extent and potential sources of racial and ethnic differences in health care. The institute formed a committee, and its findings were published in 2003. And not just as an article in an academic medical journal, but as a whole book.

It took damn near 800 pages to describe all the findings in a book entitled *Unequal Treatment: Confronting Racial and Ethnic Disparities in Health care.*[1]

Still, those within Medicine never think their direct actions, or the medical system's issues, are responsible for any health disparities. It's always about those "non-compliant" patients or just "the way that community is" that Medicine blames for poor health outcomes. The closest Medicine gets to taking responsibility is suggesting it's those *other* doctors, the bad apples, the poorly run clinics, and the inefficient hospitals "that done it."

Take Dr. Stanley Goldfarb, a former dean of an Ivy medical school and nephrologist. I'd gamble that being nephrologists is where our similarities end. He has parlayed a series of articles for the *Wall Street Journal* into a book published in March 2022: *Take Two Aspirin and Call Me by My Pronouns: Why Turning Doctors into Social Justice Warriors Is Destroying American Medicine.*[2] I couldn't bring myself to pay actual money for this book and my local libraries didn't have a copy, but between the free pages provided on Google Books and Amazon reviews, I think I got the gist of it. As the title suggests, awareness of how marginalization, race included, has shaped the country and Medicine is dismissed as "wokeism," which, in his opinion, is replacing rigorous training in the scientific basis of medical care. Goldfarb calls the assertion that racism and White supremacy contribute to racial disparities in health outcomes "crippling mythology."

Of the eight Amazon reviews posted at the time of this writing, only one gave a one-star rating, calling it completely out of touch. This reviewer was the only person who gave their full name, an Indian one. I'd bet good money that the other seven reviews, all five-star, were posted by White men. Prove me wrong.

One of these glowing reviewers was impressed that Goldfarb included solutions like this one: "If academic medical centers want to improve Black lives, they should open spacious and well-staffed outpatient facilities in inner-city neighborhoods in addition to their multimillion-dollar units placed in affluent suburbs. It may be cheaper, of course, to launch highly publicized virtue signaling anti-racist campaigns, but I suspect most Black patients would prefer good outpatient care to good intentions." As if the quality of facilities is the only issue keeping Black patients from equitable care.

A couple of chapters ago I mentioned a *JAMA Clinical Reviews* podcast by Dr. Edward Livingston, an associate editor of *JAMA*, and Dr. Mitch Katz, president and CEO of New York City Health and Hospitals, where they discussed "structural racism for skeptics."[3] Livingston believed racism became "illegal," long before Obama was elected and even before Oprah earned her first million, when civil rights legislation passed in the 1960s.

Well, Katz attempted to gently correct Livingston. Katz explained that structural racism wasn't about whether someone was a "racist" but rather how systems and policies perpetuate racial inequality. With this part, I agree, but instead of providing an example of how Medicine perpetuates racism—like, say, in all those equations where clinicians use race to make decisions about a person's care—he gave examples *outside* Medicine, such as where freeways are built and how the air pollution might affect the health of its neighbors. Not surprisingly, Dr. Skeptic took away that racial disparities were really about income and opportunity—he did not consider that Black folks had been, and continue to be, forbidden from moving out of poor neighborhoods or getting a job because they were Black. Because that would be illegal, he insisted. Therefore, he argued, the "unfortunate term" *racism* was what was really causing harm—and should be taken out of conversations of health disparities—because it offended good White folk like himself.

And the real kick in the teeth? If someone could regurgitate what they learned enough to score 80% on a test on this conversation, they could earn a continuing medical education credit toward maintaining their license to practice.

#BlackMedTwitter was outraged, me included, and we collectively went into Wonder Twins–activate mode. That took the form of tweets, emails, and meetings with AMA leadership that contributed to the podcast being taken down, Livingston resigning, and the editor-in-chief Dr. Howard Bauchner stepping down after a lame apology and attempt to smooth things over by hosting a video with a panel of respectable Black doctors.

These examples are a testament to the depths of Medicine's denial. Medicine's attitudes bear striking resemblance to society's insistence on claiming America isn't racist. Between Karen Gone Wild videos and police murdering unarmed Black people over minor traffic violations, that claim is hard to believe. Certainly, the similarities between Medicine and the larger society don't end there.

Early in my research career, I went to Jackson, Mississippi to meet with the Jackson Heart Study research team. The Jackson Heart Study is the largest single-site, community-based investigation of factors associated with cardiovascular disease in Black adults. At the time, the roughly 700 Black people in the study had been followed for five years on average and participated in D-ARIC, the dental ancillary study to ARIC, the Atherosclerosis Risk in Communities Study, a prospective community-based study of the causes and natural history of fatty deposits in arteries among adults in four US communities.[4] This mattered because my research at the time was to show if periodontal, or severe gum, disease was a risk factor for worsening chronic kidney disease. One could argue how much this research mattered in the grand scheme. It often felt silly even to me to spend hundreds of thousands of federal and philanthropic dollars on research to show having a chronic infection in one's mouth can damage the kidneys, especially when two decades of research had already shown it to be so for the heart. Still, I hoped my research would help justify providing basic dental care to the masses—something we should have always been doing. Relative importance aside, there were no other existing studies in which participants had a complete dental exam that measured the depth of gum pockets around each tooth in six specific places *and* kidney function measures at the time of dental exam and years later. So I needed to make friends with the Jackson Heart Study research team to get access to their data.

Outside my Jackson hotel window, I could see a city building proudly waving a Confederate flag—as did all the city's buildings then. Born and raised in North Carolina, it wasn't like I hadn't seen a Confederate flag on display many times before. But as someone who came of age in the 1980s, the examples were mostly in the back of a pickup truck along with a shotgun rack. A government-sanctioned display of hate hit differently. Though the few people I interacted with at the hotel or in restaurants were pleasant enough, I did not feel welcome or safe.

I asked Dr. Herman Taylor, a Black cardiologist and director of the Jackson Heart Study at the time, how the Black people in Jackson felt about the flags.

"Most people have a lot of bigger issues to be concerned about, so to them, it's just a piece of cloth," he answered.

Assuming he really heard people say that, I imagine that sentiment was more of a reflection of how Black people in Mississippi are treated. Living in the worst racial disparities in the country, they couldn't possibly have the time or energy to be offended by a flag. With so many racist battles to fight, they simply chose not to fight that one, not because the Confederate flag is just a piece of cloth—because it certainly has meaning. And it ain't that bullshit refrain about pride in Southern heritage. Now, the flag represents White supremacy, and likely always has. The Confederate flag has been appearing on lawns, truck windows, and up flagpoles far from the Mason-Dixon line—one need only recall images of Canada's "Freedom Convoy" of January 2022, in which protesters proudly waved the Confederate flag on their semi-trucks, to know better.

The Confederate flag glorifies a time when Black people were considered no more than livestock. It is used as a form of intimidation. A reminder of what has been and what could be again—as was violently demonstrated at the January 6 insurrection. No different than how the number of schools, roads, monuments at courthouses, and other government grounds memorializing Confederate veterans multiplied in number right around the time White people began violently retaliating against Reconstruction, marking the end of the 12 years immediately following the Civil War when roughly four million newly freed Black people suddenly had the right to vote and used it to elect nearly 2,000 Black people. A spike in Confederate memorials happened again during the 1950s in response to the beginnings of the Civil Rights Movement.

Just as society has its symbols that harken back to more blatantly racist times, so does Medicine. For example, the medical student dorm that opened Columbia University's Upper Manhattan campus in 1931 was named Bard

Hall as a tribute to Dr. Samuel Bard, the founder of the medical school—only the second in the country. Bard was also President George Washington's physician and delivered Alexander Hamilton's son.

He was also a slave owner.

Dr. Ray Givens learned about this history in 2016, by way of the Columbia University & Slavery project's website.[5] The project was inspired by Craig Steven Wilder's *Ebony and Ivy: Race, Slavery, and the Troubled History of America's Universities*, published in 2013.[6] Wilder's book followed the 2006 publication of *Report of the Brown University Steering Committee on Slavery and Justice*, which was commissioned by Ruth Simmons, the first Black person named as president of an Ivy League school.[7] As his book title suggests, Wilder details how slavery funded colleges, built campuses, and paid professors' salaries. For the subsequent Columbia project, Pulitzer Prize–winning history professor Eric Foner led a research seminar for undergraduate students. They presented their research to university president Lee Bollinger in the fall of 2016.

At the time, Givens, a Black man, had just transitioned from Columbia's cardiology fellowship to faculty. Since 2011 he'd lived in an apartment where he could almost spit from his kitchen window while doing the dishes and hit Bard Hall. As a fellow, Givens received the Samuel Bard Young Investigator Award from the Department of Medicine, whose chairs held the title Samuel Bard Professor of Medicine. He watched in frustration as Columbia relegated the project to publicity and fundraising—with no mention of what would be *done* about the slavery etched into the campus. He didn't feel speaking out would be a wise career choice then.

He was haunted by the images of Eric Garner being choked to death by police officers in Staten Island. Not because they were the first such images he had seen, far from it. Maybe it was because it happened just 25 miles away, or because his wife was pregnant with their first son, that this police murder affected him so deeply. There's something about bringing a child into the world that can make someone reflect on life. Weeks later, while Michael Brown laid on a Ferguson, Missouri, street hours after being murdered by a police officer, Givens was in a labor delivery room with his wife.

When his son graduated from daycare to a preschool located on the third floor of Bard Hall, his feelings around the murder of George Floyd, and Eric Garner, and all his long hours watching the disparate toll of the pandemic on Black people, boiled over and he couldn't be silent any longer.

"On the one hand, it was a point of pride to be able to give my son that type of head start in life," he said in a CNN interview. "But knowing that I was dropping him off every day in a building named for somebody who would have seen him as property was kind of a heavy feeling."[8]

He started with the Department of Medicine Chair and was met with angry disbelief and demand for proof that a professorship in honor of Bard was inappropriate. After some back and forth and pressure from hospital leadership, the professorship disappeared. But to remove Bard Hall was beyond the scope of the medical school. It was a university issue.

When he was met with similar resistance from university president Bollinger, including a demand for proof even though the project findings had been presented directly to him, Givens decided to start a petition on Change.org.

"I didn't necessarily think the petition was going to make a difference," he said. Rather, he saw it as a way to draw eyes and send the message that they can't do this in the dark.[9]

"I wanted to force honesty, transparency, and accountability—and to create a public record as insurance against retaliation, so no one could say I was suddenly bad at my job."

That fall, Bollinger announced that Bard Hall name would change because he "felt a sense of urgency."[10] But as of now, two years later, 50 Haven Avenue, New York, New York, has yet to be renamed.

In 1934, the nearly nine-foot-tall bronze statue of J. Marion Sims, "the father of gynecology," was erected on a granite pedestal at the northeastern corner of Central Park, opposite the New York Academy of Medicine. The pedestal is flanked by supporting piers, each with a stone medallion engraved in all caps. The medallion on the left reads: "Surgeon and Philanthropist, Founder of the Woman's Hospital state of New York. His brilliant achievement carried the fame of American surgery throughout the entire world." The medallion to the statue's right reads: "In recognition of his services in the cause of science and mankind. Awarded highest honors by his countrymen and decorations from the governments of Belgium, France, Italy, Spain and Portugal." Other monuments to Sims stand on the grounds of his alma mater, Jefferson Medical College, the state house in Columbia, South Carolina, and the Alabama State Capitol building in Montgomery.

Not one of these statues mentions how he tortured enslaved Black women for years. In *Medical Apartheid*, Harriet Washington provides an account of how Sims took in 11 enslaved women with vesicovaginal fistula—a devastating condition in which urine and/or stool constantly leak through an opening between the vagina and bladder and/or rectum as a result of prolonged labor through a pelvis too small for childbearing (as is common when one is forced to breed sooner than usual, as enslaved women were)—so that he could surgically experiment on them from 1845 to 1849, without all the acts that the Victorian period required to preserve the modesty of the delicate White woman, who would be examined by feel beneath massive layers of chaste skirts.[11] The enslaved women could be forced to undress completely and get on hands and knees like animals for any number of White male physicians who would repeatedly prod with a special speculum and ogle in full view what none had seen before. The enslaved women could be denied anesthesia, which was invented in 1846, and left to scream blood-curdling cries while being held down by several men as Sims tried and tried again to perfect his craft of repair over and over again—the vaginal wall tissue, quick to tear, become infected, and reopen—before he dare attempt such a thing on a White woman. The enslaved woman could become addicted to morphine—provided in large doses only after surgery—to keep her coming back for more. No, there was not one mention of how the so-called father of modern gynecology really came to hold the title on the statues erected in celebration of his great accomplishments.

Seshat Mack was among those enraged by this omission. Having grown up in Harlem, which abuts the northeastern corner of Central Park, she often walked by Sims's statue. She passed the statue daily on her commute to Mount Sinai Medical School, where she attended a joint MD/PhD program. It wasn't just part of a routine. As the daughter of physicians, she had learned from her parents the history behind the statue, and she was painfully reminded of it every time she saw it.

People in the neighborhood had been complaining about the statue for decades. But it wasn't until 2017—right after the Charlottesville Unite the Right protest—that she became part of the push to remove the statue through the Black Youth Project 100, an organization for Black people between 18 and 35 years old committed to fighting for justice and equality for Black people, that resulted in action. Four members, Jewel Cadet, Darializa Avila Chevalier, Alexis Yeboah-Kodie, and Jamila Felix, staged a dramatic protest in hospital gowns, drenched with blood over their wombs—posing a striking image that went viral.

"I don't think we could've predicted how far-reaching that image would be," Seshat said.[12]

Months later, in 2018, New York City officials voted to have the statue taken down from Central Park—and moved to Green-Wood Cemetery in Brooklyn, where Sims is buried. Still no mention of the enslaved women he tortured.

"Yeah, we don't feel great about [that outcome]," she said. "We wanted it to come down and stay down."

Seshat was the only medical person involved in the protest, but it was not for lack of effort on her part.

"I tried talking to some folks within the medical school and our diversity and inclusion departments about whether there was anything that we could do about this statue, but it never really went anywhere," she recalled.

Later, she was invited to write a blog post for the medical school about the statue's removal.

"I was kinda frustrated with that because it seemed very much like they were trying to take credit for something that they had nothing to do with after the fact," she said. "Like the person who organized this protest went to our medical school and therefore…"

Of course they did. That's what Medicine does. Or they at least try, if allowed. Seshat did not write the blog post.

As someone from a rural area, I never heard of a "county hospital" until I walked into Highland Hospital in Oakland, California, for my primary care residency interview. Yet I immediately felt I belonged. Because of the pictures. On the interview-day tour, a group of us hopefuls were led through a wide-open space to the classrooms where medical grand rounds were held. Above the entrance hung a gigantic painting of a little Black girl. She was laughing. As we were led through the classroom toward the internal medicine offices, we passed several framed 8 x 10 black-and-white pictures of prominent Black surgeons along with some White ones. There was one of Charles Drew, the founder of the first modern blood bank and one of the few Negroes prominent enough to be retained in even the Whitewashed American history books, along with Rosa Parks, MLK, and Crispus Attucks. There were also pictures of Hughenna L. Gauntlett, the first Black woman certified by the American Board of Surgery, in 1968; Daniel Hale Williams, the first Black surgeon to successfully repair a heart injury, in 1893, two years after the first American surgeon had done so; and Samuel L. Kountz, pioneering kidney transplant surgeon, who performed the first successful kidney transplant between humans who weren't identical twins.

While I suspect the pictures of surgeons, and predominantly Black surgeons at that, in the hallway leading to the Internal Medicine Department were a remnant of the tenure of Dr. Claude Organ Jr.—general surgery icon and second Black president of the American College of Surgeons—as chair of the hospital's surgical residency program from 1989 to 2003, that they are still on display, to this day, speaks to the pervading tone of the place. Either that or inertia. Regardless, this stood in sharp contrast to my days roaming the lecture halls of Duke School of Medicine. Those halls were full of large, full-color portraits of White men as far as the eye could see.

Highland Hospital felt welcoming and gave me a sense of belonging. Duke communicated that not only did I not belong, but no one who looked like me had ever done anything worthy of having a portrait commissioned, much less framed and hung on the wall.

And that is the point.

Perhaps not a conscious point—after all, the halls lined with old White men represented those who were there. Historically, Medicine excluded all Black doctor hopefuls from even walking those halls.

But being conscious or subconscious doesn't matter. Medicine is quick to point out that the intention was not to exclude or make some feel unwelcome, as if that somehow excuses the *impact*. Medicine points out intention as if it somehow lessens or negates the impact. Only corrective action can accomplish that.

This brings up another way Medicine demonstrates it reflects the racism of society: the purposeful exclusion of Black people. Just as Jim Crow laws were implemented to quell the rights that newly emancipated Black people achieved during Reconstruction, Medicine had its own set of exclusionary rules.

Jim Crow laws excluded Black people from "White" spaces and disenfranchised Black voters with poll taxes and literacy tests. Medicine closed its schools to aspiring Black doctors and its "White" hospital wards to Black patients.

The first Black doctors were educated outside the US. Dr. James McCune Smith, the first Black person to earn a medical degree, in 1837, studied at the University of Glasgow in Scotland. It wasn't until 1847 that a US medical school graduated its first Black doctor, Dr. David Jones Peck. By 1860, eight other Northern medical schools admitted Black people, but in the interim, the American Medical Association (AMA), the nation's oldest and largest physician association, had released an 1850 report that asserted "[the] Negro brain is nine cubic inches less than the Teutonic [European]," codifying the sentiment that Black people couldn't be smart enough to be doctors.[13]

Between 1868 and 1904, seven Black medical schools were established, educating the vast majority of Black doctors, 85.5% in 1905. Not only did the AMA sanction the exclusion of Black physicians as members from the day it was founded in 1847 until the 1960s—without membership, Black physicians were denied referrals, hospital admitting privileges, medical licensure, and training opportunities—it was also instrumental in shutting down Black medical schools by urging the Carnegie Foundation to commission the infamous Flexner Report.

Abraham Flexner, an American educator, conducted an in-depth evaluation of the 168 medical schools in the US and Canada that was published in 1910.[14] It's unclear how many schools closed or merged as a result of his report but by 1923 only 66 medical schools remained. And of the seven Black medical schools at the time, he believed only Meharry Medical College in Nashville, Tennessee, and Howard University College of Medicine in Washington, DC, were worthy of further development because "ten million [Negros] live in close contact with 60 million Whites," he stated. Since he considered Black people "a potential source of infection and contagion," he agreed they needed their own physicians but recommended Black physicians should be trained differently: as "sanitarians" for "hygiene rather than surgery."

And it took another act of Congress, the 1965 passage of Medicare and Medicaid programs, to force US hospitals to desegregate their wards if they wanted those federal dollars. Yet one could argue that segregated care continues within our academic institutions today, where the mostly Black and Latinx people who disproportionately make up the Medicaid population are treated by resident physicians, while the privately insured are cared for by attending physicians. See how Medicine continues the dark legacy? No racial slurs or cross-burning is needed.

CHAPTER 8

EXCEPTIONS TO THE RULE

"We all have biases." This is the mantra of every diversity, equity, and inclusion training. And everyone nods their head along in full agreement, acknowledging that, yes, we are all imperfect. We are all bound to make mistakes.

I've found that acknowledgment ends when a person's actual bias is pointed out. Then it's all White tears and pearl clutching.

Take the primary care physician colleague, a White man I had known for over a decade, who sent me a handwritten note, open and in an unsecured envelope, by way of our mutual patient's caregiver, another White man. The note could be read by the caregiver and anyone else he cared to share it with on his way to deliver it to staff in the dialysis unit who would ultimately hand the letter over to me. In the nearly four years the patient had been under my care, the colleague had not once reached out to me by email, phone, text, tweet, telegraph, smoke signal, or even a damn carrier pigeon regarding our patient.

He had, however, reached out to my boss, another White man, and a hospital executive, yet another White man, a few months prior when the White man caregiver first complained that no one in the dialysis unit was listening to him. The caregiver never spoke to me directly about his concerns because, I subsequently learned, he found me "intimidating."

The note read:

To Dialysis Clinic—Vanessa Grubbs, MD

Please ensure that [patient] receives the correct amount of chair time, with the associated anticipated weight to achieve a weight of ~52 kg. Insufficient dialysis leads to pulmonary edema; excess dialysis leads to hypotension and bradycardia. [Patient] has little room for error, as rehospitalizations are very de-stabilizing. Her last dialysis resulted [in] insufficient volume reduction of 1L and her discharged [weight] was 53.0 kg. She only received <u>one half</u> the time of active dialysis.

First, this colleague had several facts about what happened wrong, but that's beside the point of this story. Significantly, he also had his medicine wrong. Dialysis involves the removal of excess water (ultrafiltration) and waste. One can have just the removal of excess water, just the removal of waste, or the removal of both in one treatment. While insufficient removal of water may eventually result in the buildup of fluid in the lungs (pulmonary edema), and removing too much water can drop the person's blood pressure (hypotension), rapid heart rate (tachycardia) is the body's response to excess ultrafiltration, not bradycardia, or slow heart rate.

But he was most wrong about sending a note as a primary care doctor attempting to explain the pros and cons of dialysis and how to properly write a dialysis prescription to a nephrologist, a literal expert in dialysis. The hubris! The Caucasity!

On reading the note, I imagined I looked like one of those cartoon characters with steam coming from its ears and the top of its head blasting off like a rocket. My ears felt like they were on fire and my heart pounded in my chest. I don't think I had ever used the word *livid* to characterize my anger before, but at that moment, it rose to the definition.

As I read, the various ways I might handle the situation began to percolate in my mind. The possible actions scrolled before my eyes Terminator-style. (A) I could swallow the disrespect and dismiss my colleague as an asshole. (B) I could share my feelings with him in a private conversation and let it go. (C) I could bitch to a select group of friends and acquaintances. Or (D) I could inform his superiors.

I dismissed A with a quick *fuck that*. There would be no stuffing it down into that place inside me where all the slights I hadn't given voice to live. I did consider B. I even called his office. When he didn't answer, I took it as a sign that this was too egregious to handle in the dark. At that time, I didn't know how rampant such behavior was throughout the institution. I just knew light was needed.

So, I chose D—I emailed my colleague, cross-copying the chief of staff and the chief of medicine, yes, Neil Powe, with a scanned copy of the note attached. At the very least, I believed this sort of behavior needed to be documented and that my colleague needed to be reprimanded.

In his response, my colleague disagreed with my characterization of his note as unprofessional and my assertion that his action had exacerbated a difficult situation. When I asked him to consider that the caregiver, the patient's fiancé, might be manipulating the teams involved in our patient's care by telling one story to one team and a different story to another to get what he perceived as a better medical outcome, he informed me that he was "well aware of the potential for patients [and caregivers] with a diagnosis of borderline personality disorder to 'split' the health care team." I found it amusing that he was offended that I implied he missed a psychiatric maneuver when he wasn't even a psychiatrist, but he couldn't predict how I might react to his explaining dialysis to me. Later, when we met alone, I suggested he wouldn't have sent such a note had I been a White man, and he exclaimed, "I reject that!" The only thing missing was pearls for his clutching.

Admittedly, I don't know if his actions were driven by my race or my gender. I don't know how to separate the parts of myself to pinpoint exactly what drives someone else's "ism." But what I do know is all involved in the patient's care, save for the patient and me, were men, and I was the only one who wasn't White, so it didn't matter which part of me allowed a colleague to inappropriately, unprofessionally, disrespectfully engage me. Racism. Sexism. The results for me are still the same, whether he is conscious of it or not.

Ultimately, my colleague did apologize for sending the note, in part at the urgings of the chief of staff, who first accused me of "escalating" the situation and stated that she knew us both to be very fine clinicians, but not without a copious amount of explanation on how there were some kernels of justification in how he handled the situation. He was advocating for the patient, after all, and as someone with a Jew and Latinx in his family tree, he couldn't possibly be guilty of the bias I accused him of.

And because of his response and the response to my C'ing—the bitching to everyone willing to listen I did at every opportunity—a few weeks later I chose another option: E. I penned a post for my blog with a redacted image of the note, to protect the patient's identity at the encouragement of a respected friend.

Some might argue that giving such situations attention is akin to giving my power away. Instead, I should shut all this out and focus on becoming the person and professional I know myself to be. Sometimes I wish I could, but mostly I feel I have no choice but to rail against it.

I have felt negativity based on my Blackness since I was 10 years old. I remember a defining moment in my fifth/sixth-grade combination "gifted and talented" class.

The teacher, a White woman with long black hair whose name I cannot remember, had assigned the class a family tree project. We were to trace our family tree as far back as we could. As a demonstration, she presented first. Next went the sixth-grade boy with a very Greek last name. His tree had the surname "Thomas" in the recent branches.

"Oh, we must be cousins!" she exclaimed, having presented a Thomas in her family tree.

They giggled into each other's eyes.

Then it was my turn.

"My mama's maiden name is Thomas," I read from my paper and paused for reaction that never came because my potential cousins were busy looking at the floor.

Maybe no one wanted to think about the rapes of enslaved women that led to our intersecting surnames. But my 10-year-old brain, still ignorant of that history, received it as no one wanted to admit being related to me—the only little Black girl recognized as "gifted and talented" in every class from fifth grade until I graduated and matriculated into a predominantly White university, where I would repeatedly be told I was only accepted because of my Black femaleness by peers and superiors.

As a first-generation university graduate and physician who grew up poor in rural North Carolina, I've found it difficult, sometimes impossible, not to internalize the message that I didn't belong, that I didn't deserve to be there, and that maybe I was inherently less than. Yet I've been deemed so intimidating that people have gone to my boss rather than directly speaking to me for incidents that others would have had the opportunity to handle themselves.

One could argue that I've been fortunate—I have not been the victim of a BBQ Becky, a Delta flight attendant, or a police officer. But this incident and others that have happened since bother me more now than they have in the last three decades.

In my blog post, I reflected on why this incident infuriated me, saddened me, and made me feel that there is no end to this regardless of my education, income, or accomplishments, and several reasons came to mind.

1. To be profiled by a stranger is one thing, but to feel like you are being profiled by someone who has known you for more than a decade is another. You would think they would understand you based on whatever experiences they've had with you, not based on prejudice they carry around in their subconscious.

2. My primary care colleague considers himself progressive, an ally. If an "ally" is unable to accept, or even consider, that their actions may have been driven by unconscious bias, then my hopes that our society will ever overcome racism are dashed. You don't stand a chance against an enemy if this is how an ally receives you.

3. I resented that the event and subsequent gaslighting required headspace, attention, and energy that non-marginalized folks don't have to surrender. Headspace, attention, and energy that I could be giving to further honing my knowledge in nephrology or to the next scientific research article, research grant, or book.

Weeks later, it got worse when someone asked Neil Powe if he had seen my post. He read it and immediately emailed and texted me, requesting to speak with me urgently. During that conversation, he encouraged me to take down the redacted note. He expressed that even though the note was "un…pro…fession…al," slowly as if the syllables hurt his tongue, posting the note might "create unnecessary trouble for me from the hospital or even the city governance," though he had heard of no such reactions. Somehow, after months, he did not have the time to talk with my colleague about sending the note in the first place. I thanked him for his time and concern, quietly hung up, and said to no one, "I ain't taking down shit."

Powe's handling of the situation reminded me of a time when a popular physician writer spoke at our medical grand rounds several years prior. The speaker, a White woman, told a story about the dark humor we use to cope with the horrors and absurdities we see and endure in Medicine. When her story began by describing a frail, White woman in a psychiatric ER, I stiffened. The mention of the patient's race was ominous. In the speaker's story, the patient begged to be freed of the leather straps binding her wrists and ankles to the gurney so that she might go to the bathroom. As predicted, the story ended with this frail, little White woman bringing the large Black security guard standing between her and the door to the bathroom to his knees with a firm grasp of his genitals and a shout of "Hey, Nigger!"

At that moment, among the stilted laughter of the 50 or so people in the space, I looked to Powe, as the chief of medicine, one of only three Black people there and the only Black man in the room, to speak up and let the speaker and the audience know the joke was not OK. I looked to him to model how to handle this kind of situation. But he said nothing.

In my lectures, when bias comes up, I've tried to make the notion that "we all have biases" more palatable by sharing my own experience. A "see, me too" moment, if you will. I tell the story of Alexandra Garcia, who was just 20 years old when she came to me from the pediatrics nephrology clinic with urine that contained blood. It was a small amount of blood that I could see only with the help of a microscope. She also had nearly 1,000 milligrams of protein in her urine when the normal amount was 150 or less. The presumed cause was thought to be thin basement membrane disease—the same disease that caused her mother and brother to have microscopic hematuria and proteinuria. Thin basement membrane disease is caused by a defect in a type of collagen passed on in families that, as the name implies, makes the membrane covering of the kidneys' filtering units—the glomeruli—too thin to keep all the blood and almost all the protein in the body that a normal thickness membrane can. If I had to have kidney disease, this is one I would choose because people typically never progress to end-stage kidney disease, hence its other name: benign familial hematuria.

Alexandra's mother had a kidney biopsy to prove she had thin basement membrane disease, but I would continue to "presume" with Alexandra because our biopsy needle wouldn't be able to reach her kidney—she was around 300 pounds. Weight alone can increase the amount of protein in the urine, causing parts of the glomeruli to scar down to nonfunctional nubbins, so her prognosis probably would not be as great as if she had thin basement membrane disease alone.

It didn't matter because the treatment was the same: an ACE inhibitor. Angiotensin-converting enzyme inhibitors are a class of blood pressure medications that are especially good at lowering the blood pressure within the kidneys, so the filters' holes have a chance to heal and allow less protein to pass through. She was already taking a small dose of an ACE inhibitor prescribed by her pediatric nephrologist. My job was to advise her to lose weight and increase the ACE inhibitor dose until the protein in her urine was less than 300 mg unless she became dizzy from low blood pressure first.

Around a year later, despite visits to the clinic every three months, the amount of protein in her urine was the same. This was in part because her weight had not decreased, and she wasn't taking her ACE inhibitor every day as prescribed.

"What's going on, Miss Garcia?" I asked. Maybe she was having trouble remembering to take it or was experiencing a dry cough, a common side effect of ACE inhibitors.

"I don't know," she giggled. "Sometimes I think the medicine kinda makes me a little tired." She giggled again.

She giggled like a little girl, not like the young woman she was. And my patience for a giggly little girl who couldn't give me a legitimate reason for not taking care of herself had worn thin.

"OK, I'm gonna need you to put on your big-girl panties and do what you know you need to do to take care of your kidneys," I lectured her and sent her on her way with a prescription for an ARB, an angiotensin II receptor blocker, as a replacement for the ACE. The ARB would work similarly and hopefully would not make her "kinda tired."

Two weeks later, I got an email from her primary care doctor with a gentle reminder that we all needed to be more diligent in our ensuring our female patients of childbearing age are using effective birth control when we prescribe ACE inhibitors and ARBs. It is well-known that ACEs and ARBs can cause birth defects. Apparently, Miss Garcia told her primary care doctor that she was only sometimes taking her medicine because her period was late.

My heart dropped.

I could try to tell myself it didn't occur to me to counsel Miss Garcia about birth control at every visit, as I did with every other woman of childbearing age I'd cared for when prescribing ACEs and ARBs, because she came to me already on an ACE or even because of her childlike demeanor. But the truth is, it hadn't occurred to me that she was sexually active because she was so large.

I've long argued that Medicine is not immune to biases because all humans have biases, conscious and unconscious. Biases that can limit our thinking. Biases that can bring harm to our patients. Biases that we need to check for when we find ourselves deviating from "standard care." I had failed to take my own advice. All I could do was learn my lesson and do better next time and all the times after that. I had to teach myself to see the full person living in every body, no matter their shape or size.

The next time I saw Miss Garcia, I apologized for not counseling her properly, but I didn't have the courage to tell her why. And maybe the tension that comes with admitting bias while looking someone in the eye is the reason most of us avoid acknowledging the pain we've caused. Doing so would mean questioning the ego we've built. We behave as if one admission of misstep would upend our whole sense of self. But in truth, I think honesty would only make us stronger.

Miss Garcia told me her unborn baby looked normal on ultrasound. I can only hope that when her baby was born the ultrasound was right.

CHAPTER 9

LACK OF PROFESSIONALISM

That one time when Uchenna Inodum (name changed for her protection) tried CBD oil in her tea in hopes of finding a natural means of silencing her PTSD anxiety, she had no idea how much it would affect her life months later. Days into starting her new family medicine residency as the only Black person in an all-White hospital (save for one janitor) in a small Northeast town, she learned that the hair sample they required was positive for THC. Program leadership didn't care that THC is legal in the state, that her urine was free of drug metabolites, nor her reason for using the oil that one time. She had to be taught a lesson.

In order to return to work, she had to participate in a drug rehab program and submit multiple urine tests. Since returning to work, she was required to submit weekly urine samples, and should even one sample come back positive, she would be fired—with six-figure debt from medical school and no license to practice medicine. She was called randomly and told to submit samples within 15 minutes of request. Never mind two of the tests were in the same week. Never mind the written policy stated one must submit their sample within an hour, not 15 minutes. Never mind this lesson worsened her anxiety and interfered with her job. She had to be taught a lesson.

"Wow, that's crazy!" a White woman peer remarked when Uchenna told her of what she was going through, then shared her own story.

Though her urine had been positive for opiates, the White peer had a very different experience. When program leadership asked for an explanation, she offered that she had jaw surgery months prior and was still having pain. Leadership thought that was reasonable, and that was the end of it. No operation report or valid prescription needed. Her word sufficed.

"And to think, I even snorted cocaine to celebrate matching!" the peer giggled. Good thing the match—when graduating medical students learn about which, if any program, has accepted them into their program—was just beyond the 90-day limit for how long hair holds evidence of drug use. But even then, that too could have been forgiven as easily as Trump's "locker room talk." She was celebrating, after all!

The point is not whether it's the program's business to monitor what someone does with substances, legal or not, on their own damn time if it doesn't harm anyone else or show up on the job. The point is not even to argue if Uchenna or the White woman was being truthful or not. I am highlighting how two women's violations of the same policy were handled differently by the same leadership.

Uchenna's story reminds me of who is believed without question. How no one asked Carolyn Bryant, who later admitted she lied, "Are you sure he whistled at you? Are you sure he said something vulgar to you?" Instead, two White men immediately beat, shot, and disfigured beyond recognition the body of 14-year-old Emmett Till in 1955. The story made me think about how in 1994, for nine days, the national media broadcast Susan Smith pleading for the safe return of her toddlers, whom she claimed a Black man kidnapped as part of a carjacking. On the tenth day, she confessed to killing them. It also made me think about how Amy Cooper had not doubted that she would be believed and that police would be deployed when she dialed 911 to falsely accuse a Black man of attacking her in a New York City birdwatching park in 2020.

According to the ACLU, sentences imposed on Black men in the federal system are nearly 20% longer than those imposed on White men convicted of similar crimes. Black people are 20 times more likely to be sentenced to life without parole for a nonviolent crime than White people.[1] According to a 2023 report from the US Department of Education's Office for Civil Rights, Black boys and girls are nearly twice as likely to receive out-of-school suspension or expulsion than their White counterparts.[2]

Medicine is no different. According to unpublished 2015–2016 data from the Accreditation Council for Graduate Medical Education, only 5% of Medicine's resident physicians were Black, but they accounted for 20% of dismissals from training programs.[3]

STAT published journalist Usha McFarling's piece entitled "'It Was Stolen from Me': Black Doctors Are Forced Out of Training Programs at Far Higher Rates Than White Residents," in June 2022.[4] Soon after, dozens of comments and social media posts immediately chimed in with a similar sentiment: "Black residents are disproportionately fired; at some point, affirmative action runs out, and the substandard simply can't cut it anymore." Some commenters backed up their assertions with figures showing that Black students had lower MCAT scores than White ones. Setting aside the fact that there are at least four more standardized tests after the MCAT, which is just used to get into medical school, on the path to being a board-certified physician. Even still, high test scores do not automatically prove that someone will make an excellent doctor. Our stories are the evidence.

Our stories say that Black medical students and physicians are judged by a different standard at every level. This demonstrates that Medicine was designed for White, cisgendered, heterosexual, slender, able-bodied, Christian men from families in the middle class and up. The closer you fit the description of who Medicine was designed for, the less traumatic and toxic it will be. The rest of us are just trying to make it through by "getting in where we fit in." Failure to fit in enough, as judged by the powers that be, will get you get pushed out, commonly under the "lack of professionalism" umbrella. "Lack of professionalism" is the new "Not a good fit," which was always code for "insufficient code-switching," so nobody has to say "Because you're Black."

And it's all by design.

In 1999, the Accreditation Council for Graduate Medical Education (ACGME) selected and endorsed a set of six core competencies to help establish the basic skills and attributes that practicing physicians should be able to demonstrate in order to graduate and excel in the field of medicine.[5]

The six vague, subjective, and easily weaponized against anyone Medicine chooses ACGME Core Competencies are as follows:

- **Practice-Based Learning and Improvement:** Demonstrates the ability to investigate and evaluate patient care practices, and appraises and assimilates scientific evidence to continuously improve patient care based on constant self-evaluation and life-long learning.

- **Patient Care and Procedural Skills:** Provides compassionate, appropriate, and effective patient care for the treatment of health problems and the promotion of health.

- **Systems-Based Practice:** Demonstrates awareness of and responsiveness to the larger context and system of health care and the ability to effectively call on other resources in the system to provide optimal health care.

- **Medical Knowledge:** Demonstrates knowledge about established and evolving biomedical, clinical, epidemiological, and social behavioral sciences as well as the application to patient care.

- **Interpersonal and Communication Skills:** Demonstrates interpersonal and communication skills that result in effective information exchange and collaboration with patients, their families, and health professionals.

- **Professionalism:** Demonstrates a commitment to carrying out professional responsibilities, and adherence to ethical principles.

Case in point: Dr. Gislaine Bernabe. Before I knew the 5%/20% data point, I knew Gislaine. We entered one another's lives virtually on November 14, 2021, just two days after a colleague from an informal Twitter community of Black physicians sounded the alarm for anyone available to help with their mentee in trouble. Several of us answered the call and assembled like the Avengers.

Born in Haiti, Gislaine immigrated to the US as a child and became a US citizen and the first in her family to graduate from college and medical school. She returned to the Caribbean for medical school for financial reasons, though many of her clinical rotations were completed in the States.

On July 1, 2021, she started working as an intern physician in a newly formed family medicine residency program at a for-profit hospital in Nashville, Tennessee, where she was one of only two international medical graduates and the only Black intern among her peers across three new training programs.

Although the Educational Commission for Foreign Medical Graduates (ECFMG) certified her as ready to enter US training programs, she found her entire career in jeopardy within the first month of her training. Instead of the program applying for her license to practice as they did all their other trainees, program leadership decided to create a narrative that she was unprofessional and incompetent and placed her on remediation with a performance improvement plan (PIP) three weeks into her internship—an action essentially unheard of so early in training. Nobody knows what they are doing in their first month out of medical school. It's frightening that one day you're wearing a short white coat of powerlessness and the very next day your signature on an order is all that's required to make something happen.

Gislaine recalls her program director responding in derisive dismay that Gislaine did not know how to order an echocardiogram in this new hospital system she had just entered days earlier. The director reacted like Gislaine told her she couldn't tie her shoes! Her most serious offense was an occasional noun-verb disagreement in her clinical notes. I say, not bad for someone fluent in four languages. I have never seen a phrase like "they was" result in a bad patient outcome. Even though Gislaine exceeded all required tasks outlined in her PIP, her remediation was escalated to probation in December 2021. Ultimately, she was terminated on January 14, 2022, for failing to meet five of six competency areas, without the hospital communicating specific reasons. With the stain of termination on her record, she was unable to successfully match into another program. She could not even "scramble" into a program with unfilled positions at the end of the formal matching process. Like many young Black residents in her position, Gislaine was facing the reality that she would be unable to work as a physician *and* that she was in debt to the tune of around $240,000. The entire experience stripped her of her confidence and joy.

Luckily, through the behind-the-scenes networking of our small group, she was able to find a new position in New York. Though she had to start over, she was thrilled to have another opportunity. As of this writing, she is not only surviving but is thriving; she was named chief resident, a designation reserved for top residents. And to think, her first program tried to throw away a brilliant doctor over some typos. A whole doctor, when according to the Association of American Medical Colleges, the United States is projected to face a shortage of up to 86,000 physicians over the next decade.[6]

It never fails that, when we tell our stories as Usha McFarling did in her article, people like the program director come out of the woodwork and say, "But where's the data," reiterating that our word is not enough. To them, I say, *"Now what, bitches?"* as I slam my data on the table like the card that sets your opponent in a contentious game of bid whist.

The data I'm referring to come from the Institutional Review Board (IRB)–approved National Study of Resident Physicians' Disciplinary Experiences I led with the help of an independent research firm and generous funding from the California Health Care Foundation and the Commonwealth Fund.[7] The study was conducted between May and August 2024, and we are preparing reports for publication in various venues. Participants were in residency programs represented by the Committee of Interns and Residents (CIR), the largest union of resident physicians, with nearly 30,000 members at the time of this study. Over 19,000 were residents (and not fellows), and 1,755 (9%) completed the study survey. Participants represented nearly all specialties, with internal medicine (20%) and family medicine (10%) most common. I think only radiation oncology was not represented. A third of survey participants identified as Asian American/Pacific Islander (34.2%), 29.7% as White, 12.3% as Hispanic/Latinx, and 10.9% as Black. I also conducted

50 in-depth individual interviews that prioritized sampling all racial/ethnic groups. Although there are 150,000 residents nationally, this is the first study of this size and richness. Most studies of this type get only about 2% response, to this one's 9%. The major limitation of the study is that we could only reach active residents, so any residents who were already dismissed would be missed.

Still, 3% of survey respondents and 6% of Black residents reported being on remediation or probation. Overall, 21% of survey respondents had been asked to meet with their program director due to negative comments from peers or faculty; 30% of Black residents had this experience. Nearly half of residents (48%) felt the negative feedback was unjustified, with 37% believing that race and 50% that gender influenced the negative feedback. Disturbingly, only 35% of residents who received negative comments reported the feedback was ever discussed with them before going to their program director. It is this going to the program director that starts the negative spotlight that leads to negative discipline experiences and is usually unquestioned.

Said one interview participant who identified as Black and had been terminated from their program shortly after completing the survey:

> I would say they take the words of attendings 100%. Literally whatever they said was written in stone. Whatever I said didn't make sense. That is how I was being treated and that hurt a lot. The attending can pretty much write whatever they want to. They can say things that are not true; they will take it for granted because they are an attending. They supposedly are doing these evaluations for a long time. They know how to write evaluations, so their word is truth 100%. Whatever they are saying, that is true. That is the impression that leadership gave me. . . . Whatever the attending said, that is the law of the land pretty much which is really unfair I feel like. I felt like there were comments on there that if you feel like this comment is true, we will go talk with the patient. We will call the patient. We have their number. Did this stuff really happen? They would not even take that step to even do that.

The resident went on to say that in their two years in the program, no patients in their care were involved in a morbidity and mortality conference, or M&M, where medical/surgical errors are dissected to understand root causes.

"They were so hard on me. There were many patients that other residents saw that led to an M&M or led to some sort of fatal outcome for patients and they let them progress into residency," they said. The other residents were White.

"What do you think you'll do now?" I asked.

"I think this is going to be one of the most challenging moments in life," they said. "Eventually, God willing, my goal is I want to get into a residency program. I want to graduate from residency."

My heart broke for this resident, and all I could do was hope that someone would give them a fair chance like Gislaine. Still, what was particularly sad about Gislaine's situation was that her program director, the one with the power to decide to escalate the situation or train Gislaine like all the other residents, was a Black woman. Somehow this fact, according to the lawyer we secured for Gislaine by crowdfunding his retainer fee, made it virtually impossible to prove she was being discriminated against because of her race or gender.

News flash, Black people can be anti-Black too. They, too, can serve to protect the system and their spot in it. I had to learn the *all skin folk ain't kin folk* lesson the hard way.

In the introduction, I told the story that made me leave academia, but I omitted the most hurtful part. How wrong I was to think that I was safe. I knew Black people in high places. In the end, not one of them spoke up on my behalf. Instead, the chief of medicine, my research mentor of 10 years, chose to escalate the situation. The chair of epidemiology and biostatistics literally ran away from me—ducked out of a group meeting before I could make it across the room to chat with them and then ignored emails and texts. And the dean who I had explicitly asked to protect me when, not if, I got in trouble over my writing, remained silent.

But it's not entirely their fault. Medicine selects for the type of Black I called "prototypical minority faculty" in my "Diversity, Equity, and Inclusion That Matter" piece. Colloquially known as respectable Negroes, these are the ones Medicine places in leadership positions because they know they will settle for micro-incremental change rather than upset the White establishment or disrupt their paycheck. The problem is, they lull Black junior faculty and trainees into a false belief that a leader will support them when issues involving race arise.

What my experience demonstrates is that the over-policing of Black physicians never ends. As I wrote in my perspective "Racism in Academic Medicine Is Hindering Progress Toward Health Equity" for the California Health Care Foundation blog, Dr. Aysha Khoury, a Black internist and faculty member at Kaiser Permanente School of Medicine (KPSOM) in Pasadena, facilitated a discussion about race and gender health bias with a small group of students in KPSOM's inaugural class in August 2020.[8] Within hours, the medical school suspended Khoury from teaching and clinical responsibilities. After an eight-week probe, during which all the students in that small group petitioned for her reinstatement, the administration dismissed Khoury. The school told her the firing was a consequence of poor clinical and teaching performance, not racism. Never racism.

Khoury, who said she was never told what policy she violated, sued the school. "My career with Kaiser is over now because the dean, the executive leadership, and the board all okayed my dismissal," said Khoury in an interview on June 22, 2021. "They gave students a primer on how to discriminate and get away with it." The National Labor Relations Board (NLRB) concluded that her claim that KPSOM's action violated the National Labor Relations Act was meritorious and filed its own separate complaint.[9]

On January 10, 2023, Khoury and KPSOM jointly announced the settlement of the civil case and the NLRB proceeding. "The settlement includes a demonstrable commitment by the school to conduct further examination of its practices relating to diversity, equity, inclusion, and implicit bias in medical education and to enhance those practices as well as share learning to positively influence medical education overall," the joint statement said.

Khoury is now a faculty member at the Morehouse School of Medicine in Atlanta.

In California, Dr. Omondi Nyong'o, a pediatric ophthalmologist in Palo Alto, and several other Black physicians have lodged complaints and filed lawsuits against Sutter Health, alleging racial discrimination at the large Sacramento-based nonprofit health system. A Sutter spokesperson issued a statement: "We deny having taken or participated in any discriminatory or retaliatory conduct against Dr. Nyong'o or any of our physician partners or our own employees."

In Louisiana, Dr. Princess Dennar, the Tulane University School of Medicine's first and only Black woman residency program director, was suspended from her job soon after filing a race discrimination lawsuit against the school. The case was settled in December 2021, and the parties have made no public comments since.

Dr. Uché Blackstock wrote an article in *STAT* about "toxic and oppressive" conditions that prompted her to leave a faculty position in an academic medical center.[10] She described more details in her 2024 book *Legacy: A Black Physician Reckons with Racism in Medicine*, including how her tweets in response to a fellow Harvard alum lamenting "prior luminaries of medicine & surgery" no longer gracing the walls of the auditorium made the powers that be very upset.[11] Her tweet pointed out how the wall represented a history of "racism, white privilege, white supremacy and sexism." Hmm, a Black woman got in trouble over a truthful tweet. Sounds so familiar.

PART IV
FROM NEGLIGENT TO CONSCIENTIOUS

CHAPTER 10

PLACEBO

Placebo is defined as "a harmless pill, medicine, or procedure prescribed more for the psychological benefit to the patient rather than for any physiological effect."[1] Once upon a time, a placebo was considered an acceptable way to give the healthy hypochondriac something to make them feel better or to use in research studies to make sure the real pill, medicine, or procedure was better than just the suggestion that this thing will make you better. But then we got the Codes of Ethics dictating standards for health care and research studies, and all of that had to stop.

Perhaps since the Los Angeles riots after the acquittal of Rodney King's attackers, Medicine has engaged in some form of placebo treatment toward its negligence problem: from the stereotypical do's and don'ts of cultural competency of old—as in, Do speak in short, simple sentences with African American patients, and Don't touch a Hmong child on the head—to the latest volunteer DEI committees and implicit bias training where participants leave owning no personal responsibility because they've never tried anything like touching a Black woman's hair. All of this has served as a psychological benefit to those with power more than any physiological benefit to those without it. But Medicine's placebo is anything but "harmless." Black people are dying at rates disproportionate to any other group on Medicine's watch, and there are no Codes of Ethics to correct it.

Not to say that the principles of diversity, equity, and inclusion aren't valid. They absolutely are. But the ways that Medicine chooses to engage with these ideas are superficial and negligent at the same time. Medicine's goal is to check off boxes and feel good about doing so.

As I pointed out in my perspective for the California Health Care Foundation blog, "diversity" has broadened to "all diversity matters," enabling institutions to lump together counts of women and non-White physicians and trainees to project a progressive façade.[2] That way, no one has to feel bad about the dearth of Black and Indigenous people in the space. Hence the term *BIPOC*—Black, Indigenous, and people of color. Medicine is very heavy on the POC, where all the Asian groups are counted, but sorely lacking the BI. Women are thrown in to make it sound better. As in, look how diverse we are, we are 50% women, even if the group is predominantly White. Medicine never fails to brag about its racial diversity in the institution overall, but fails to mention that the vast majority of that BI diversity is concentrated among the janitorial and cafeteria staff. They are missing in the C-suite, except maybe for the occasional "respectable Negro."

For example, the 2015 American Hospital Association "Diversity and Disparities" report examined diversity within US hospitals, focusing on gaps between frontline staff diversity and leadership.[3] It found that while over half of hospital staff are women and a significant portion come from racial-minority backgrounds, only about 11% of hospital executive leaders and 14% of board members were people of color.[4] The 2021 joint report by the American Medical Association and the Association of American Medical Colleges, "Advancing Health Equity: A Guide to Language, Narrative, and Concepts," discusses the impact of leadership diversity on health equity, pointing out that although minority representation among medical students and residents has increased, hospital and health system executives remain predominantly White and male. The report found that systemic barriers in health care, such as a lack of leadership development programs and mentorship for minorities, contribute to this gap.[5] While many US health care organizations employed a diverse clinical workforce, their C-suites and boards lack comparable diversity. In other words,

Black employees are significantly underrepresented in decision-making roles, despite health care's diverse patient base.

One only needs to look at pay disparities to know that Medicine does not value "equity." There has been a notable lack of Black physician advancement in academic medical institutions, and pay disparities have been well documented. According to a 2021 report from the Association of American Medical Colleges, only 3% of academic medical school full professors are Black women, and only 1.7% are Black men. Among clinical science department chairs, only 1.8% are Black women and 2.8% are Black men. Among physician faculty, for every dollar a White man is paid, on average a Black man is paid 93 cents, a White woman 77 cents, and a Black woman 73 cents.[6]

"Inclusion" is supposed to make a person feel valued, involved, and respected for the viewpoints, ideas, perspectives, and experiences they bring. But Medicine's version of inclusion is expected service on committees, panels, and boards on diversity, equity, and inclusion, only to have their voice drowned out by the majority or more powerful perspective. Further, this version of inclusion equates to what is known as a "minority tax" that impedes career advancement. This service is usually uncompensated and contributes to a façade. It is a time commitment not expected of White colleagues, who stay focused on activities that lead to promotions, including research and publication.

Medicine chronically undervalues Black physicians. A study examining applications for federal health research grants found Black researchers' applications submitted between fiscal years 2000 and 2006 were more likely to be overlooked, less likely to be considered fundable, and focused on topics with lower award rates.[7] The irony of this finding is that after George Floyd's murder, well-funded scientists who are White and have relatively little background in health equity research are disproportionately being awarded grants in that field. Their scientific endeavors often build on the research of Black and Latinx scholars without citing them or offering to include them on grants or as coauthors.[8]

Dr. Camara Jones, who I've dubbed "Queen of the Allegory" and whose Gardener's Tale allegory I described earlier in the book, likens Medicine's behavior to a potluck. "It's like they feel as if they're sitting at a potluck," she says.[9] "They see you come in, and they don't want you anywhere near the table because they think you're going to come eat up all the food. . . . They don't see that you're bringing all kinds of cakes, and pies, and roasts."

She goes on to describe the impact. "It is a loss of our genius that saps the strength of the whole society. The loss is not recognized because people think that they have everybody at the table that they need without us. They don't value us."

Probably the worst implicit bias training I've ever been a part of happened as part of the California Health Care Foundation Health Care Leadership Fellowship. Launched in 2001, "this two-year, part-time fellowship offers clinically trained health care professionals the experience and skills necessary for effective vision and leadership in the health care system."[10] The fellowship is known for being life-changing, with many fellows literally changing jobs during the program. I certainly fit that mold as I made the decision to leave UCSF during the fellowship.

I was part of Cohort 18, also known as the bitter cohort because the pandemic stripped us of the real graduation experience. Participation required two in-person two-day meetings each year with monthly small group, aka pod, meetings in between. There were only three Black people in our cohort, and I was the only Black woman. Because the three of us lived or worked in Oakland or San Francisco, we were all in the same pod, along with three Asian colleagues and one White woman who we jokingly referred to as our token White woman.

During our last pre-Rona (the time before the coronavirus took over the planet) in-person gathering, they broke us up into two groups of 16 for some of the sessions. One of the sessions was the DEI portion of the fellowship, which the facilitator called "Building Bridges." The facilitator, a Native Hawaiian man, stressed the importance of finding common ground with others, even with those who might have diametrically opposed views and politics. This was, he said, "being in pono," a Hawaiian phrase meaning "to be in a state of harmony or balance with oneself, others, the land, work, and life itself."

He then took us through an exercise in which we rotated around the room into triads. He would pose a question for one person to answer for one minute while the other two just listened. The other two were to thank them for sharing and offer no commentary before rotating into their next triad.

And this is where it goes left, like a sordid joke told at a dinner party: So, a Jewish woman, a Black woman, and a middle-aged White woman enter a triad.

"For the next minute, tell the story of when you first became aware of your race," said the facilitator.

The middle-aged White woman was up to speak. "Umm, I don't know how to answer this question," she stuttered. "I was just always raised not to see color and I believe that if I were to go for a job interview everybody has the same chance of getting it."

I blinked hard in disbelief. I knew that all of California was not the liberal mecca some make it out to be. One doesn't have to drive far outside of San Francisco to find die-hard Trump supporters. And then there are the NIMBYs of places like Berkeley, where people are thought to be very liberal until you try to build low-income housing in their neighborhoods. Then it's "Not in My Back Yard!" The middle-aged White woman was from Bakersfield. For those unfamiliar with California geography, Bakersfield is at the southern end of the San Joaquin Valley. When I first moved to California, I learned the area is referred to as the "Armpit of California" because, according to the Urban Dictionary, oil refineries pollute the dry, desert air, and there are more cows than people. Bakersfield also tops the list of most conservative cities in California and makes the top 10 list of most conservative cities in the country. But still, I thought my fellowship peers were developed, thoughtful health care professionals. That moment, and all the related moments after, taught me how truly naïve I was.

"Thank you for sharing," I mustered when I really wanted to say, "Bitch, what?!" The Jewish woman muttered her thank you and we both rotated away like the good little rule-followers we were asked to be in that moment. There was no room to unpack any of the words she said or the feelings they prompted. I felt saying nothing allowed Bakersfield to walk away with the belief the problematic thing she said was ok.

But I didn't let it go. Couldn't let it go. I talked to others. Turns out, the other half of the cohort weren't good rule-followers and forced a conversation.

I gave honest feedback in the written evaluation. The facilitator asked to speak with me. I explained why the interaction was problematic.

And then the real placebo effect happened.

At the next meeting, which was virtual, thanks to the pandemic, I was set up. This was our final meeting and would conclude with our graduation. I suppose I could have kept quiet as the facilitator shared a video depicting a White actor saying almost verbatim what Bakersfield said. But I'm more of an address-the-elephant-in-the-room type of person, and my peers who knew of the situation were prodding me with direct messages in the Zoom chat.

I shared with the class what it felt like for someone to say they didn't see color when I was in the thick of people treating me differently because of my color. How it felt to be so painfully aware of how people perceived me because of my color, while a White person got to walk through life never really having to consider theirs. I said everything short of calling out Bakersfield by name. Being so honest was painful. I ugly-cried, hoping to be heard and validated through my tears and cracking voice.

But in the end, I felt that none of my words mattered. When the other woman in that triad got involved and slipped up by calling Bakersfield by name, Bakersfield became visibly upset. Many people in the fellowship ultimately defaulted to comforting her because that is how our society, Medicine included, responds to a White woman in tears.

We've seen it repeatedly. In 2020, we all saw Amy Cooper become increasingly distressed in Central Park while she claimed that Christian Cooper, the Black man recording her, was threatening her when all he really did was ask her to leash her dog so he could bird-watch. In 2018, we saw Jennifer Schulte, aka BBQ Becky, become visibly emotional when a bystander questioned her depiction of Black men trying to grill some chicken and burgers at Lake Merritt park.

In Medicine, it looks like White medical students, nurses, and physicians characterizing their interactions with Black peers as intimidating or aggressive. When issues of race arise, White people displaying defensiveness and tears evokes sympathy from instructors and administrators, which derails any uncomfortable conversation and any progress.

In this case, the conversation about implicit racism was overtaken by Bakersfield's emotional reaction. She was so upset that she threatened to quit the fellowship, the day of graduation.

I don't know what was said behind the scenes, but Bakersfield was convinced to come back, but she was excused from participating in our "Essence" session, where everybody else shared something that showed who they believed themselves to be at their core. Somebody shared a video. Some wrote letters. I shared poems I had written during medical school and residency, including "Stranded," which opens this book. It was emotional. There were a lot of tears. But Bakersfield was protected.

In the last moments of this virtual meeting, we were all asked to say something we learned from our experience.

"I think it's better that I don't speak right now," I said. "I'm really upset."

"Well, we'll come back to you, but everyone has to share," the Black woman faculty member leading the conversation told me.

I was not Bakersfield. I was not to be protected. I was a Black woman. I am reminded of Malcolm X's words, "The most disrespected person in America is the Black woman. The most unprotected person in America is the Black woman. The most neglected person in America is the Black woman."[11]

"I learned that I need to be more careful with some of the things I say," said Bakersfield.

And when it got back to me, I said, "I learned that White pain is more important than mine."

I noticed one of my peers of color roll her eyes.

CHAPTER 11

HUMILITY

There is, sadly, no magic pill to cure Medicine's negligent behaviors. It will require work and humility. Cultural humility because cultural competence is not good enough.

The Drs. Melanie Tervalon and Jann Murray-García explain what the work of cultural humility ought to look like in their article "Cultural Humility Versus Cultural Competence: A Critical Distinction in Defining Physician Training Outcomes in Multicultural Education," published in the *Journal of Health Care for the Poor and Underserved* in May 1998.[1] In my mind, these two trailblazing Black woman physicians have earned their *The* for creating the concept of "cultural humility" alone.

I first met Melanie when I was attempting to bring the tenets of cultural humility to Highland Hospital, where I stayed on as faculty after completing my residency. As I wrote in my first book, *Hundreds of Interlaced Fingers*, I reached out to her for help. At the time, Melanie was in her early fifties. She walked into the room with a certain regality, with her shoulder-length, straightened, blond-silver hair and her chin tilted up just so. But maybe that was just how I saw her, the legend in my mind, as an international figure in the work and for her medical school class valedictorian speech calling out institutional racism. I have been honored to be a friend to her—and even credit her with bringing my husband and me together.

Recently, more than 20 years after that first meeting, I sat beside her on her navy-blue chenille sofa. Her hair is all silver now, worn short in her natural, soft curls. Golden-yellow walls dotted with artist friends' work surrounded us, telltale signs of a bold woman's living room. Dr. Murray-García filled the screen of my laptop.

It was my first meeting with Jann, albeit virtual, and the fangirling was real. I was stunned to hear her say she was a fan of *my* work. I had wanted to meet with them to learn the context behind theirs.

Like everything, it starts with how one is raised.

Melanie grew up in the Civil Rights Movement and integrated Philadelphia schools. "I knew very deeply what it meant to be the only Black person in these small Catholic private schools and on through the whole education process," she said. Raised in a family with three siblings, she often heard one of them share a story about being treated horribly, and her parents would pack them all up and head back to the school immediately to handle it. Each event ended with her father reiterating that they were not inferior to White people. She and her siblings grew up *knowing* that the notion of White supremacy was simply ridiculous. She went on to work with the Third World Women's Alliance, the Angela Davis Defense Committee, and the Black Panther Party Clinic, *before* her famed medical school graduation address.

"These deep ties to community and community organizing was really in my heart, in my spirit, in my body, in my being, and in my intellectual processes, when it came time to be, when we were presented with what happened at Children's [Hospital of Oakland in the wake of the Rodney King riots in Los Angeles] and thus birthed that cultural humility process."

Jann, on the other hand, came from teacher parents who were deeply politically involved in the communities where they lived, most recently East San Jose, California. She was very grounded in the history of her ancestors. She told me her maternal grandfather was an African Methodist Episcopal pastor in South Carolina. He graduated from Boston University in 1923, earned a master's degree in 1924, and went on to teach Greek, Hebrew, and theology at Allen University, a historically Black college in Columbia, South Carolina.

He later became the president of the NAACP in Charleston in the 1940s and 1950s, a role that often led to getting beat up.

"But what I heard from my mom, just woven in as she was a brilliant teacher, was that he said that he would never see these changes, that he was working for his children and his grandchildren. And so, every time I get tired, I think about that. Like Maya Angelou said, I am that dream," Jann said. "So, I have this sense that what we do matters."

In their article, Melanie and Jann make the case for committing to a lifelong learner model, because one can never fully know the nuances of a group they don't belong to, and attempting to do so from a cultural competence model of do's and don'ts opens us up to mistreating patients when the "teachings" simply aren't true. It's one thing to be aware of the Southeast Asian healing practice of "coining" so as not to accuse the parents of a Cambodian child with the characteristic linear marking, they argue, but another thing altogether for a nurse to "know" that "Hispanic patients overexpress the pain they are feeling." In the latter case described, the nurse's presumed expertise stereotyped the patient's experience and led her to ignore the moaning patient just out of surgery in front of her. In this way, one must be flexible and humble enough to acknowledge what they do not know and adopt an honest process of self-critique and self-awareness to challenge their own attitudes toward people from different backgrounds.

Cultural humility also entails redressing the power imbalances in the physician-patient dynamic. Melanie and Jann challenge the clinician to recognize the expertise that the patient brings to the encounter when it comes to communicating across culture. Because, for example, it is only the Mexican American, male, father, husband, Catholic, mechanic, night-school student and resident of East Los Angeles—not the doctor—who is qualified to help the doctor understand how the intersections of race, ethnicity, religion, class, et cetera form his identity and clarify how it all relates to and impacts his present illness or wellness experience. This requires patient-focused interviewing, which is a less controlling, less authoritative style that lets the patient know that the clinician values the patient's agenda and perspectives and allows the patient to be a capable and full partner in the therapeutic alliance.

Finally, cultural humility requires developing mutually beneficial and non-paternalistic partnerships with communities on behalf of individuals and defined populations. Here, Melanie and Jann are urging clinical training to take place in community sites—where most physicians ultimately practice— and away from the university-based, largely subspecialized medical centers. This requires an acknowledgment that physician responsibility should extend beyond individual patient care to advocacy within the community to change policies and practices that drive the determinants of health, causes of disease, and the efficacy of health care provision.

This is a far cry from my experience. When I was applying to internal medicine residency programs shortly after this paper came out, before I knew it existed, programs in Northern California were calling an extra half-day per week clinic in one's third year a "primary care track." That's how hospital-centric training was then, and a large part of why I ended up at Highland Hospital in Oakland for residency. The primary care track felt like much more than an afterthought, but still I remember a resident giving the applicant tour telling me what wonderful "pathology" they were exposed to there. Translation: "There is so little access to primary preventive care for poor people in this community, we get to see all the really advanced cases. And we like it like this."

So when I asked Melanie and Jann how they were able to gain traction to move the work forward, they told me about countless hours of meetings, organizing, learning personal details to connect with individuals in power, and making specific asks.

Publishing the work was another hurdle. Years passed with only a pile of rejections to show for it.

"I remember Jann calling me one morning and saying everybody's rejecting the paper and the last group that wanted to publish it said, oh we'll publish it if you take out that line that talks about race and gender and/or whatever in there, and I said, well, if that comes out there's nothing left in there," said Melanie.

At that point, Melanie was prepared to forgo academic publishing. But Jann persisted.

"Let me try one more place," Jann had said.

That place was the *Journal of Health Care for the Poor and Underserved*, founded in 1990 by Dr. David Satcher, America's first Black surgeon general. The journal published the article as it was written.

Yet publishing was not the end goal. It was just a means of spreading the concept. Ultimately, the goal was liberation, Melanie declared.

Melanie described how, a couple of years later, she was attending a conference on culture. The presenter wanted everyone to play a board game on cultural competence.

"And it was just truly, horrifically stereotypic," Melanie recalled. "I was horrified, and I was sitting there thinking I have to say something, and I don't know what I'm going say, when a young White woman in the audience shot up her hand and blasted the presenter."

"Do you know nothing about cultural humility?" that woman said and ran down Melanie and Jann's paper. Verbatim. Melanie watched in stunned amazement.

In the years since, both Melanie and Jann have been training people in the model of cultural humility. The people have covered the gamut, from community organizers to heads of hospitals and everyone in the health sector between. They have trained thousands of people. Thousands who have gone on to take it back to their institutions and organizations and trained more people.

"I had no idea that this was how this was going to emerge and how it would be taken by people as being so important to them and so transformative," Melanie said. "Until I think as maybe a decade after it was published, people would be writing to me, and to Jann, with these similar ideas of saying, I read it and I realized that's what I always believed and I'd never seen it before, you know. So that's when I understood how carrying this back to the community organizing piece connected with the fact that when we wrote it, we saw ourselves into writing with the voice of the community."

Make no mistake, neither Melanie nor Jann believe cultural humility has turned Medicine around. But they do believe, they know for sure, that they have made a contribution.

"I have this sense that generations from now, there will be this turn in an appreciation in what cultural humility has to offer for people," said Melanie.

CONCLUSION

REALITY

At the time of this writing, it's been more than a quarter of a century since Drs. Tervalon and Murray-García wrote about cultural humility. Let's face it. Medicine ain't trying to hear about self-reflection and lifelong learning, at least when it comes to Black people: be it a patient, trainee, or practicing clinician. In large part, because cultural humility requires sitting with—and never fully mastering or becoming "competent" in—issues like identity, power, and history.

That whole "racial reckoning" following the murder of George Floyd came and went. Though they were little more than placebo, DEI programs and committees have all but dried up in the face of anti-DEI legislation around the country.

At the time of this writing, convicted felon Donald J. Trump has been reelected, presumably democratically, when the other option was an uber-qualified Black and South Asian woman. Another reminder that racism and misogynoir are real and consequential. And this is the way of history. For every step forward we take, *they* do everything they can to push us back at least three-quarters of that step. As Frederick Douglass said way back in 1857, "Power concedes nothing without a demand. It never did and it never will."[1]

But what I do know is that we continue to move forward. I hesitate to call it "progress," as I am reminded of Malcolm X's words, "If you stick a knife in my back nine inches and pull it out six inches, there's no progress. If you pull it all the way out, that's not progress. The progress is healing the wound that the blow made . . . And they won't even admit the knife is there."[2]

Progress would be liberation for all. Liberation for me would be feeling like I could watch my son leave home in the morning and expect him to return safely later, even if he was stopped for a routine traffic check. Still, we have moved forward. Chattel slavery has been abolished. Granted, it has been replaced with mass incarceration and prison labor, which makes it "forward," not "progress." I often think about how Congressman John "Good Trouble" Lewis fought his entire life for the right to vote but lay on his deathbed writing an opinion piece urging us to keep fighting. All while we watched his efforts, and the work of so many others, be undone.

In Medicine, progress would be health care for all. A step forward was the 1964 passage of Title VI of the Civil Rights Act, which withheld federal funding from any hospital that refused to desegregate. Progress has been impeded, however, by health care that allows for a new kind of segregation between private and public insurance. Progress would be for everyone with the ability, desire, and wherewithal to become a doctor having the opportunity to do so. So while Black people are admitted to medical schools, where medical training should be a safe place to learn from our mistakes, we have instead a hidden curriculum of an implicit but distinct set of rules for success, as well as a *haunted* curriculum. In their 2024 article in *Medical Education* entitled "When I Say . . . Haunted Curriculum," which uplifted the work of Black and Indigenous scholars, Dr. Jennifer Karlin and her colleagues describe how forms of oppression and injustice are always present in training, a lurking presence that demands change but is too often denied. "Like ghosts, not everyone sees these forms of oppression, and not everyone believes those who do."[3]

So how do we demand? How do we address the anti-Blackness in American Medicine? How do we transition Medicine from negligent to conscientious, even in the face of opposition?

The opinions on how to heal Medicine are abundant, resulting in multiple factions. We don't have time to wait for all of us to get on the same page, because lives are literally at stake.

And the thing is, we don't all have to take the same approach, because the elephant in the room is huge. We don't all have to take a bite out of its ass at once. We can gather around it and just get to chewing.

We can organize.

Medical students showed us how to with their efforts to end race correction for kidney function. Usha Lee McFarling and Katie Palmer captured just how much work it took in their piece "Inside the Bruising Battle to Purge Race from a Kidney Disease Calculator" published by *STAT* in 2024.[4] After interviewing dozens of kidney specialists, including me, they wrote about the contentious battle, much of which I sensed but did not experience firsthand. It was a true David and Goliath ordeal, but in the end, a race-free equation was published in 2021.[5] Since then, the other race-based algorithms have been falling like dominos. And there will be no going back.

We can create organizations for us.

"We've got to stop allowing them to push our young doctors out," I said to the small group of Black physicians who gathered around Gislaine Bernabe. And that was the beginning of Black Doc Village, the 501(c)(3) nonprofit organization I founded in April 2022. While I imagine the name may scare off some people, understand the name was intentional. We are intentional about our vision: a future where the training of Black physicians is prioritized, celebrated, and supported as a cornerstone of addressing physician workforce concerns, improving health outcomes for the Black community, and moving closer toward realizing health equity broadly speaking. This vision is built on a foundation of strategic partnerships, alternative program approaches, policy advocacy, data-driven storytelling, and meaningful investment, all aimed at dismantling long-standing barriers and fostering an environment where Black physicians thrive.

This intention has allowed us in the last year to carry out work that the huge, long-standing, well-funded organizations haven't or won't conduct to bring tangible data, partially detailed earlier in the book, to paint the picture of what some of us already knew. With these data and more to come, we will press forward toward the vision we seek.

I started with the same modus operandi as other organizations, trying to support individuals like Gislaine who found themselves under the negative spotlight. I reasoned like the African proverb; it would take a village to raise the next generation of Black doctors. But then the inner primary care doctor who believes in prevention took over. Don't get me wrong, helping those in trouble is important work, and at some point, we have to figure out how to prevent our young people from falling off the metaphorical cliff and push them back from the ledge, out of harm's way. Here, I'm reminded again of Dr. Camara Jones and her allegory on how to address the social determinants of health. One might notice some people living close to the cliff's edge, frequently falling off and sustaining tragic injuries from which most succumb. One might respond by building a state-of-the-art hospital to tend to those who survive quickly and efficiently. One might erect a net partway up the cliff's edge to help minimize the severity of injuries. Or one might turn their attention to changing the circumstances that historically put those on edge and in harm's way. The approach of Black Doc Village recognizes that other small organizations trying to catch folks teetering on the edge are dependent upon the "free" time of many people. I'm a believer that one of the many functions of White supremacy is to keep us all too busy, so we don't have enough time to get the things done that pay the bills, much less have time left over to do all the social justice work we might want to do.

Through Black Doc Village, we plan to leverage our data into policy change, such as mandating the Centers for Medicare and Medicaid Services (the primary investor in medical residency training) to collect data to ensure that the billions of federal taxpayer dollars ($16.2 billion in 2021 alone) directed to graduate medical education every year are creating the diverse physician workforce it's been charged to build. Maybe we can leverage our data into policy change that will change how the money is distributed so that programs are reminded that the funding is to train *all* the young doctors in their program, not disproportionately discard the Black ones because they were deemed to not be a "good fit." Perhaps we can use these data to leverage our change into conferences like morbidity and mortality conferences, except for equity, where instead of faculty, staff, and sometimes peers making negative claims that are automatically taken as truth, they are investigated and looked at from all sides.

If you'd like to be a part of this effort, join us. Give money. Help build the grassroots movement that we've started. But if my approach doesn't tickle your fancy, that's okay too, because again, the elephant is huge. Bite where you feel the most change will happen because at the end of the day, we need to eat the whole goddamn elephant—as Black Southerners say about the pig—from the rooter to the tooter. But whatever you do, don't interfere with our efforts. Stand on the sidelines and cheer, but don't throw tacks and barbs in our path as we try to run, because you disagree or want limelight to yourself.

We can rebuild our own safe spaces.

Shortly after the 1910 publication of the damning Flexner Report, five of the nation's seven Black medical schools, unable to finance required facility and training upgrades, shut down. Until the 1920s, more than 500 Black hospitals were intricately linked to the medical training programs that provided essential training grounds for Black doctors.[6] With the loss of these institutions, we are left with a system that dismisses Black resident physicians at four times their representation. This century-long absence has contributed to persistent health inequities within the Black community. These institutions were not merely educational facilities but vital community hubs that fostered cultural concordance—the shared identity between patients and health care providers.

The need for cultural concordance in health care is often misunderstood or misrepresented as segregation rather than being recognized as a crucial element in delivering equitable care. Cultural concordance is crucial because it significantly improves health outcomes. Emerging literature now underscores the importance of training health care professionals from diverse communities. It is increasingly clear that institutions must intentionally produce culturally concordant health care providers who can understand and address their communities' unique needs. This is not just a matter of fairness or representation, but a proven strategy for improving health outcomes and achieving health equity.

Baywell Health, formerly West Oakland Health, has a vision to do just that. During the Black Power and Civil Rights Movements, four Black mothers—Jessie Hamilton, Edith Brown, Olivia Parks, and Cloteal Davis—saw a need and took action. With the help of state funding and nearly 30 volunteer Black doctors, they launched West Oakland Health Council and opened its doors in March 1967.

I walked through those doors and started seeing patients in March 2023. I wrote about my experience in an article, "The Gift I Didn't Realize I Needed," for the California Health Care Foundation blog in 2024.[7] It was the gift I didn't realize I needed, because I came for the vision articulated by new leadership (including my husband Robert Phillips, president and CEO) to be an unapologetically Black-led, Black-serving, and Black-focused organization striving to be a hub for the health and dignity of the Bay Area's Black community. I didn't expect to be able to be my full, authentic, un-code-switched self there.

On my first Saturday clinic, I found Black women at registration, a Black woman nurse, and a Black woman medical assistant. I not only felt a sense of joy, I also felt comfortable chanting "Black lady clinic! [*clap clap*], Black lady clinic! [*clap clap*]" à la the courtroom segment on *A Black Lady Sketch Show*. I have since greeted these coworkers and others who frequently sport new braids, faux locs, weaves, or hair colors with, "OK, hair!" They return a smile and perhaps a flip of their new hair without having to block the hand of someone trying to touch their hair or having to answer the tiresome question "*How much of that is yours?*" because the answer is always, "All of it because I have the receipt," followed by a "And no, you can't touch it."

It looked like me pointing out a need, proposing a solution, and being encouraged by open-minded leadership to develop it—so much so that I recently was named director of adult medicine. It didn't work this way in the predominantly White institutions where I worked. In those organizations, I was repeatedly tokenized to meet the diversity requirement on unpaid committees whose majorities drowned out my voice or tone-policed me for being too direct.

When I saw White patients in predominantly White institutions, I often felt a bit on edge, as if I had to prove myself. It was an anticipatory reaction to all the times White patients had asked me where I went to medical school. As nonchalantly as possible, I would say "Duke" to back them down. But it didn't matter where I went to school—I still had to pass all the same board certification examinations as everybody else. At best, I figured, they were going to think of me as "different" from other Black people, at worst inherently inadequate because I was Black. At Baywell Health, patients don't ask where I went to medical school. No one assumes I've gotten where I am today because of affirmative action, because everyone knows the adage about Black people having to work twice as hard to get half as much.

While I know my Duke degrees (both undergraduate and medical) opened doors for me, if I had a do-over, I would spend my entire education in predominantly Black spaces like historically Black colleges and universities, free of the "you're only here because you're a Black female" accusations. I didn't know any better the first time around due to the misconceptions that afflicts many of us. I was raised by blue-collar parents from Alabama who were born in the early 1930s; I was brought up to believe that the White man's ice is indeed colder. Believing that everything White is automatically superior is internalized racism. That belief left me chasing the approval of Whiteness to validate my worth and find a sense of belonging. Admittedly, it's easy to fall into the trap of seeing reality as those in power shape it to be. I'm reminded of how in my small writing group's effort to publish "Genomic Supremacy: The Harm of Conflating Genetic Ancestry and Race," we started with the highest impact journals and went down the list, rejection by rejection.[8] The impact factor is a metric that reflects how often a journal's articles are cited over the last two years to suggest its relative importance. Journals with higher impact factor values are considered more important and prestigious in the field.

Finally, after nine rejections, I said, "You know, this is part of how White supremacy works. They decide which journals have the highest impact. They control what is published." The journals that rejected us suggested we send the paper to the *Journal of Health Care for the Poor and Underserved*, a publication they have deemed as lesser. That idea was tacitly shut down and the article ended up in the *Human Genomics* journal in May 2022. Now I will be starting with the *Journal of Health Care for the Poor and Underserved* when I begin to formally publish Black Doc Village's findings. Those in power should not decide who and what is worth publishing based on race.

I even feel smarter at a predominantly Black institution, because at the clinic I sense my intelligence is assumed, not questioned. When I enter an exam room to greet a White patient (of course we take care of everyone who comes in), I don't feel that edge here. By walking through the doors of Baywell Health, the patient has demonstrated they have no objection to me being Black. At the clinic, my non-Black colleagues (we have those too) have demonstrated the humility needed to care for a predominantly Black population and embrace our mission to center Black people.

But even in this space, I've unfortunately encountered people who bring the same bullshit from predominantly White institutions. Again, I'm learning that all self-proclaimed allies aren't accomplices and all skin folk ain't kin folk. Some so-called allies have the appearance of being good, until their power is challenged. Then they pull the reverse racism card. To them I say, "No, Boo Boo," I'm not challenging your opiate policy because you're a White man, it's because I refuse to allow you to make my 80-year-old patient pee in a cup every month because she needs one Tylenol with codeine every night to quiet her grating knees enough to rest. Some skin folk are all about the community until you touch an insecure nerve. Then it's damn near "fuck them kids." To them I say, Boo Boo, I am not your enemy just because I disagree with you.

I ended my piece for the CHCF blog paraphrasing a prolific poet of our time: "We got 99 problems, but—unlike our predominantly White counterparts—being Black ain't one." However, I never thought I'd find pretend allies and non-kinfolk to be 2 of the 99 in this space. Bless my naïve heart yet again. I am well into my fifties and still learning that, given the opportunity, "people gonna people" no matter the cause at stake. But thankfully, at Baywell Health, a Black-led health center, the only remaining predominantly Black-serving federally qualified health center in California, my voice—unlike at predominantly White institutions I have experienced—is heard and valued.

And like I tell my patients who want to know if I'm planning to stay, "I ain't going nowhere." Just like all the Black women trailblazers who came before me, I will persist because the abolition of anti-Blackness in Medicine requires that I do.

And yet, in this moment, I am wondering exactly who "we" is. I hope it can be us.

NOTES

INTRODUCTION
NEGLIGENT MEDICINE

1 Vanessa Grubbs, *Hundreds of Interlaced Fingers: A Kidney Doctor's Search for the Perfect Match* (Amistad, 2017).

2 *Merriam-Webster*, s.v. "negligence," accessed November 24, 2024, www.merriam-webster.com/dictionary/negligence.

3 Audre Lorde, *The Master's Tools Will Never Dismantle the Master's House* (Penguin Classics, 2018).

CHAPTER 1
RACE SCIENCE

1 Emily S. Renschler and Janet Monge, "The Samuel George Morton Cranial Collection: Historical Significance and New Research," *Expedition Magazine* 50, no. 3 (November 2008), www.penn.museum/sites/expedition/the-samuel-george-morton-cranial-collection.

2 Josiah C. Nott and George R. Gliddon, *Types of Mankind: or, Ethnological researches based upon the ancient monuments, paintings, sculptures, and crania of races, and upon their natural, geographical, philological and Biblical history: Illustrated by selections from the inedited papers of Samuel George Morton and by additional contributions from L. Agassiz, W. Usher, and H. S. Patterson* (Philadelphia: J. B. Lippincott, Grambo & Co., 1854), www.loc.gov/item/49043133.

3 Theresa Overfield, *Biological Variations in Health and Illness: Race, Age, and Sex Differences*, 2nd ed. (CRC, 1995).

4 Thomas Jefferson, "Query XIV: The Law," in *Notes on the State of Virginia* (London: John Stockdale, 1787), www.monticello.org/thomas-jefferson /thomas-jefferson-and/notes-on-the-state-of-virginia/notes-on-the-state -of-virginia-query-xiv.

5 Samuel Cartwright, "Report on the Diseases and Physical Peculiarities of the Negro Race," *New Orleans Medical and Surgical Journal*, 1851.

6 Harriet A. Washington, *Medical Apartheid: The Dark History of Medical Experimentation on Black Americans from Colonial Times to the Present* (Doubleday, 2006).

7 Ken Belson, "Black Former NFL Players Say Racial Bias Skews Concussion Payouts," *New York Times*, August 25, 2020, www.nytimes.com/2020 /08/25/sports/football/nfl-concussion-racial-bias.html.

8 Marc A. Norman, David J. Moore, Michael Taylor, Donald Franklin Jr., Lucette Cysique, Chris Ake, et al., "Demographically Corrected Norms for African Americans and Caucasians on the Hopkins Verbal Learning Test-Revised, Brief Visuospatial Memory Test-Revised, Stroop Color and Word Test, and Wisconsin Card Sorting Test 64-Card Version," *Journal of Clinical and Experimental Neuropsychology* 33, no. 7 (2011): 793–804, https://pmc.ncbi.nlm.nih.gov/articles/PMC3154384/.

9 John Brown, *Slave Life in Georgia: A Narrative of the Life, Sufferings, and Escape of John Brown, a Fugitive Slave, Now in England,* ed. Louis Alexis Chamerovzow, (London: W. M. Watts, 1855), www.docsouth.unc.edu /neh/jbrown/jbrown.html

10 Washington, *Medical Apartheid*, 58.

11 K. L. Clay, "Despite the Odds: Unpacking the Politics of Black Resilience Neoliberalism," *American Educational Research Journal* 56, no. 1 (February 2019): 75–110, https://doi.org/10.3102/0002831218790214.

12 D. A. Vyas, D. S. Jones, A. R. Meadows, K. Diouf, N. M. Nour, and J. Schantz-Dunn, "Challenging the Use of Race in the Vaginal Birth after Cesarean Section Calculator," *Women's Health Issues* 29, no. 3 (May–June 2019): 201–4, https://doi.org/10.1016/j.whi.2019.04.007.

13 Rolanda L. Lister, Wonder Drake, Baldwin H. Scott, and Cornelia Graves, "Black Maternal Mortality-The Elephant in the Room," *World Journal of Gynecology and Women's Health* 3, no. 1 (2019), https://doi.org/10.33552/wjgwh.2019.03.000555.

14 William P. Chapman and Chester M. Jones, "Variations in Cutaneous and Visceral Pain Sensitivity in Normal Subjects," *Journal of Clinical Investigation* 23, no. 1 (January 1944): 81–91, https://doi.org/10.1172/JCI101475

15 Kelly M. Hoffman, Sophie Trawalter, Jordan R. Axt, and M. Norman Oliver, "Racial Bias in Pain Assessment and Treatment Recommendations, and False Beliefs About Biological Differences Between Blacks and Whites," *Proceedings of the National Academy of Sciences* 113, no. 16 (April, 2016): 4296–301, https://doi.org/10.1073/pnas.1516047113.

16 I. Bavli and D. S. Jones, "Race Correction and the X-Ray Machine—The Controversy over Increased Radiation Doses for Black Americans in 1968," *New England Journal of Medicine* 387, no. 10 (September 2022): 947–52, https://doi.org/10.1056/NEJMms2206281.

17 J. Larry Jameson, Anthony Fauci, Dennis Kasper, Stephen Hauser, Dan Longo, and Joseph Loscalzo, *Harrison's Manual of Medicine* (McGraw Hill, 2020).

18 Sripal Bangalore, Yan Gong, Rhonda M. Cooper-DeHoff, Carl J. Pepine, and Franz H. Messerli, "2014 Eighth Joint National Committee Panel Recommendation for Blood Pressure Targets Revisited," *Journal of the American College of Cardiology* 64, no. 8 (August 2014): 784–93, https://doi.org/10.1016/j.jacc.2014.05.044.

19 Osagie K. Obasogie, "Oprah's Unhealthy Mistake," *Los Angeles Times*, May 17, 2007, www.latimes.com/archives/la-xpm-2007-may-17-oe-obasogie17-story.html.

20 Cartwright, "Report on the Diseases."

21 Lundy Braun, *Breathing Race into the Machine: The Surprising Career of the Spirometer from Plantation to Genetics* (University of Minnesota Press, 2014).

22 R. Kumar, M. A. Seibold, M. C. Aldrich, L. K. Williams, A. P. Reiner, L. Colangelo, et al., "Genetic Ancestry in Lung-Function Predictions," *New England Journal of Medicine* 363, no. 4 (July 2010): 321–30, https://doi.org/10.1056/NEJMoa0907897.

23 Duana Fullwiley, "The Biologistical Construction of Race," *Social Studies of Science* 38, no. 5 (October 2008): 695–735, https://doi.org/10.1177/0306312708090796.

CHAPTER 2
LOW-HANGING FRUIT

1 Andrew S. Levey, "A More Accurate Method to Estimate Glomerular Filtration Rate from Serum Creatinine: A New Prediction Equation," *Annals of Internal Medicine* 130, no. 6 (March 1999): 461, https://doi.org/10.7326/0003-4819-130-6-199903160-00002.

2 Modification of Diet in Renal Disease Study Group, Lawrence G. Hunsicker, Sharon Adler, Arlene Caggiula, Brian K. England, Tom Greene, et al., "Predictors of the Progression of Renal Disease in the Modification of Diet in Renal Disease Study," *Kidney International* 51, no. 6 (June 1997): 1908–19, https://doi.org/10.1038/ki.1997.260.

3 David W. Harsha, Ralph R. Frerichs, and Gerald S. Berenson, "Densitometry and Anthropometry of Black and White Children," *Human Biology* 50, no. 3 (1978), https://digitalcommons.wayne.edu/humbiol/vol50/iss3/6.

4 S. H. Cohn, C. Abesamis, I. Zanzi, J. F. Aloia, S. Yasumura, and K. J. Ellis, "Body Elemental Composition: Comparison Between Black and White Adults," *American Journal of Physiology-Endocrinology and Metabolism* 232, no. 4 (April 1977), https://doi.org/10.1152/ajpendo.1977.232.4.e419.

5 J. G. Worrall, V. Phongsathorn, R. J. Hooper, and Elisabeth W. Paice, "Racial Variation in Serum Creatine Kinase Unrelated to Lean Body Mass," *Rheumatology* 29, no. 5 (1990): 371–73, https://doi.org/10.1093/rheumatology/29.5.371.

6 Harsha et al., "Densitometry."

7 "Previous EGFR Calculator for Reference," National Institute of Diabetes and Digestive and Kidney Diseases, 2009, www.niddk.nih.gov/health-information/professionals/clinical-tools-patient-management/kidney-disease/laboratory-evaluation/estimated-gfr-calculators/previous.

8 Andrew S. Levey, Lesley A. Stevens, Christopher H. Schmid, Yaping (Lucy) Zhang, Alejandro F. Castro III, Harold I. Feldman, et al., "A New Equation to Estimate Glomerular Filtration Rate," *Annals of Internal Medicine* 150, no. 9 (2009): 604–12, https://doi.org/10.7326/0003-4819-150-9-200905050-00006.

9 Lesley A. Inker, Christopher H. Schmid, Hocine Tighiouart, John H. Eckfeldt, Harold I. Feldman, Tom Greene, et al., "Estimating Glomerular Filtration Rate from Serum Creatinine and Cystatin C," *New England Journal of Medicine* 367, no. 21 (July, 2012): 20–29, https://doi.org/10.1056/NEJMoa1114248.

10 Dorothy Roberts, "The Problem with Race-Based Medicine," TEDMED Talk, February 12, 2016, www.tedmed.com/talks/show?id=530900.

11 C. Delgado, M. Baweja, N. R. Burrows, D. C. Crews, N. D. Eneanya, C. A. Gadegbeku, et al., "Reassessing the Inclusion of Race in Diagnosing Kidney Diseases: An Interim Report from the NKF-ASN Task Force," *Journal of the American Society of Nephrology* 32, no. 6 (2021): 1305–3017, https://doi.org/10.1681/asn.2021070988.

12 Sibel Yucel Kocak and Arzu Ozdemir, "Comparison of Creatinine, Cystatin, CKD-EPI Cystatin C, CKD-EPI Creatinine and MDRD Equations in Estimating Glomerular Filtration Rate in Patients with Nephrotic Syndrome," *Cumhuriyet Medical Journal* 43, no. 2 (May 2021): 155–56, https://doi.org/10.7197/cmj.909706.

13 Roni Caryn Rabin, "A 'Race-Free' Approach to Diagnosing Kidney Disease," *New York Times*, September 23, 2021, www.nytimes.com/2021/09/23/health/kidney-disease-black-patients.html.

14 Jessica P. Cerdeña, Jennifer Tsai, and Vanessa Grubbs, "APOL1, Black Race, and Kidney Disease: Turning Attention to Structural Racism," *American Journal of Kidney Disease* 77, no. 6 (2021): 857–60, https://doi.org/10.1053/j.ajkd.2020.11.029.

15 Krista L. Lentine, Bertram L. Kasiske, Andrew S. Levey, Patricia L. Adams, Josefina Alberú, Mohamed A. Bakr, et al., "KDIGO Clinical Practice Guideline on the Evaluation and Care of Living Kidney Donors," *Transplantation* 101, no. 8S (August 2017), https://doi.org/10.1097/tp .0000000000001769.

CHAPTER 3
THE SEARCH CONTINUES

1 Supinda Bunyavanich, Chantal Grant, and Alfin Vicencio, "Racial/Ethnic Variation in Nasal Gene Expression of Transmembrane Serine Protease 2 (TMPRSS2)," *JAMA* 324, no. 15 (October 2020): 1567, https://doi.org /10.1001/jama.2020.17386.

2 Priya Vart, Niels Jongs, David C. Wheeler, Hiddo J. Heerspink, Anna Maria Langkilde, and Glenn M. Chertow, "Effectiveness and Safety of Dapagliflozin for Black and White Patients with Chronic Kidney Disease in North and South America," *JAMA Network Open* 6, no. 4 (April 2023), https://doi.org/10.1001/jamanetworkopen.2023.10877.

3 Vart et al., "Effectiveness and Safety of Dapagliflozin."

4 Nancy E. Adler and David H. Rehkopf, "U.S. Disparities in Health: Descriptions, Causes, and Mechanisms," *Annual Review of Public Health* 29, (April 2008): 235–52, https://doi.org/10.1146/annurev.publhealth .29.020907.090852.

5 Alastair J. J. Wood, "Racial Differences in the Response to Drugs—Pointers to Genetic Differences," *New England Journal of Medicine* 344, no. 18 (May 2001): 1394–96, https://doi.org/10.1056/nejm200105033441811.

6 C. W. Yancy, M. Fowler, and W. S. Colucci, "Race and the Response to Adrenergic Blockade with Carvedilol in Patients with Chronic Heart Failure," *ACC Current Journal Review* 10, no. 5 (September 2001): 52, https://doi.org/10.1016/s1062-1458(01)00392-0.

7 D. V. Exner, D. L. Dries, M. J. Domanski, and J. N. Cohn, "Lesser Response to Angiotensin-Converting-Enzyme Inhibitor Therapy in Black

as Compared with White Patients with Left Ventricular Dysfunction," *ACC Current Journal Review* 10, no. 5 (September 2001): 51, https://doi .org/10.1016/s1062-1458(01)00390-7.

8 Vanessa Grubbs, "Precision in GFR Reporting: Let's Stop Playing the Race Card," *Clinical Journal of the American Society of Nephrology* 15, no. 8 (August 2020): 1201–2, https://doi.org/10.2215/cjn.00690120.

9 Camille E. Powe, Michele K. Evans, Julia Wenger, Alan B. Zonderman, Anders H. Berg, Michael Nalls, et al., "Vitamin D–Binding Protein and Vitamin D Status of Black Americans and White Americans," *New England Journal of Medicine* 369, no. 21 (November 2013): 1991–2000, https://doi.org/10.1056/nejmoa1306357.

10 "Antihypertensive and Lipid-Lowering Treatment to Prevent Heart Attack Trial (ALLHAT)," National Heart Lung and Blood Institute, n.d., accessed November 12, 2024, www.nhlbi.nih.gov/science/antihypertensive -and-lipid-lowering-treatment-prevent-heart-attack-trial-allhat.

11 The ALLHAT Officers and Coordinators for the ALLHAT Collaborative Research Group, "Major Outcomes in High-Risk Hypertensive Patients Randomized to Angiotensin-Converting Enzyme Inhibitor or Calcium Channel Blocker vs Diuretic: The Antihypertensive and Lipid-Lowering Treatment to Prevent Heart Attack Trial (ALLHAT)," *JAMA* 288, no. 23 (December 2002): 2981–97, https://doi.org/10.1001/jama.288.23.2981.

12 Vart et al., "Dapagliflozin for Black and White Patients."

13 Robert S. Schwartz, "Racial Profiling in Medical Research," *New England Journal of Medicine* 344, no. 18 (May 2001): 1392–93, https://doi. org/10.1056/nejm200105033441810.

14 Jessica P. Cerdeña, Vanessa Grubbs, and Amy L. Non, "Racialising Genetic Risk: Assumptions, Realities, and Recommendations," *Lancet* 400, no. 10368 (December 2022): 2147–54, https://doi.org/10.1016 /s0140-6736(22)02040-2; Jessica P. Cerdeña, Vanessa Grubbs, and Amy L. Non, "Genomic Supremacy: The Harm of Conflating Genetic Ancestry and Race," *Human Genomics* 16, no. 18 (May 2022), https://doi.org /10.1186/s40246-022-00391-2; Vanessa Grubbs, Jessica P. Cerdeña, and

Amy L. Non, "The Misuse of Race in the Search for Disease-Causing Alleles." *Lancet* 399, no. 10330 (March 2022): 1110–11, https://doi.org /10.1016/s0140-6736(22)00488-3.

15 Camara P. Jones, "Levels of Racism: A Theoretic Framework and a Gardener's Tale," *American Journal of Public Health* 90, no. 8 (August 2000): 1212–15, https://doi.org/10.2105/ajph.90.8.1212.

CHAPTER 4
MELANIN AND LOCKS

1 Vanessa Grubbs, "California Dermatologists Offer Equitable Care to Dark-Skinned Patients," California Health Care Foundation, March 25, 2021, www.chcf.org/blog/california-dermatologists-offer-equitable-care -dark-skinned-patients.

2 Roni Caryn Rabin, "Dermatology Has a Problem with Skin Color," *New York Times*, August 30, 2020, www.nytimes.com/2020/08/30/health/skin -diseases-black-hispanic.html.

3 David T. Robles and Daniel Berg, "Abnormal Wound Healing: Keloids," *Clinics in Dermatology* 25, no. 1 (January 2007): 26–32, https://doi.org /10.1016/j.clindermatol.2006.09.009.

4 "Pathology Central: Race in Medicine," YouTube playlist by Pathology Central, accessed November 13, 2024, www.youtube.com/playlist?list =PLTeFWuy4f0bSdYMOAoQPA4CUksMUHncqH.

5 Vinay Kumar, Abul K. Abbas, and Jon C. Aster, eds., *Robbins Basic Pathology* ill. James A. Perkins, 10th ed. (Elsevier, 2018).

6 Robles and Berg, "Abnormal Wound Healing."

7 Anthony E. Brissett and David A. Sherris, "Scar Contractures, Hypertrophic Scars, and Keloids," *Facial Plastic Surgery* 17, no. 4 (2001): 263–72, https://doi.org/10.1055/s-2001-18827; Syed M. Alhady and K. Sivanantharajah, "Keloids in Various Races: A Review of 175 Cases," *Plastic and Reconstructive Surgery* 44, no. 6 (December 1969): 564–66, https://doi.org /10.1097/00006534-196912000-00006.

8 Edward A. Kitlowski, "The Treatment of Keloids and Keloidal Scars," *Plastic and Reconstructive Surgery* 12, no. 6 (December 1953): 383–91, https://doi.org/10.1097/00006534-195312000-00001; J. C. Allan and P. Keen, "The Management of Keloid in the South African Bantu," *South African Medical Journal* 28, no. 49 (1954): 1034–37, https://pubmed.ncbi.nlm.nih.gov/13216369.

9 Tayfun Aköz, Kaan Gideroğlu, and Mithat Akan, "Combination of Different Techniques for the Treatment of Earlobe Keloids," *Aesthetic Plastic Surgery* 26 (May 2002): 184–88, https://doi.org/10.1007/s00266-002-1490-3.

10 B. Cosman, G. F. Crikelair, D. M. C. Ju, J. C. Gaulin, and R. Lattes, "The Surgical Treatment of Keloids," *Plastic and Reconstructive Surgery* 27, no. 4 (April 1961): 335–58, https://doi.org/10.1097/00006534-196104000-00001.

11 Cosman et al., "Surgical Treatment of Keloids."

12 T. Naegeli, "Recherches statistiques, expérimentales et biologiques sur les chéloides," *Bulletin de la Société française de dermatologie et de syphiligraphie* 38 (1931): 905; Staub, "In discussion, Lespinnes: Tatouages en reliefs et chéloïdes des chez nègre du Congo," *Bulletin de la Société française de dermatologie et de syphiligraphie* 38 (1931): 927.

13 A. J. Koonin, "The Aetiology of Keloids: A Review of the Literature and a New Hypothesis," *South African Medical Journal* 38 (November 1964): 913–16, https://journals.co.za/doi/pdf/10.10520/AJA20785135_43567.

14 I. C. LeFlore, "Misconceptions Regarding Elective Plastic Surgery in the Black Patient," *Journal of the National Medical Association* 72, no. 10 (October 1980): 947–48, https://pmc.ncbi.nlm.nih.gov/articles/PMC2552534.

15 Michael W. Sjoding, Robert P. Dickson, Theodore J. Iwashyna, Steven E. Gay, and Thomas S. Valley, "Racial Bias in Pulse Oximetry Measurement," *New England Journal of Medicine* 383, no. 25 (December 2020): 2477–78, https://doi.org/10.1056/nejmc2029240.

16 Vanessa Grubbs, "The Health Care System Has the Black Community in a Choke Hold," California Health Care Foundation, August 4, 2020, www.chcf.org/blog/health-care-system-has-black-community-choke-hold.

17 Shannon Sabo and Sandra Johnson, "Males and the Hispanic, American Indian and Alaska Native Populations Experienced Disproportionate Increases in Deaths During Pandemic," US Census Bureau, June 22, 2023, www.census.gov/library/stories/2023/06/covid-19-impacts-on -mortality-by-race-ethnicity-and-sex.html.

18 "Pulse Oximeters," US Food and Drug Administration, last updated January 6, 2025, www.fda.gov/medical-devices/products-and-medical -procedures/pulse-oximeters.

CHAPTER 5
BLACK VOICES UNHEARD

1 American Society of Bioethics and Humanities, *Core Competencies in Healthcare Ethics Consultation*, 2nd ed. (American Society of Bioethics and Humanities, 2011).

2 Austin Frakt and Toni Monkovic, "A 'Rare Case Where Racial Biases' Protected African-Americans," New York Times, November 25, 2019, www .nytimes.com/2019/11/25/upshot/opioid-epidemic-blacks.html.

3 John Thomas, Calvin Calhoun, Con O. T. Ball, R. S. Anderson, and George R. Meneely, "Acute Myocardial Infarction in Ninety Negro Patients: Clinical Manifestations and Immediate Mortality: Comparison with 229 Similarly Studied White Patients," American Journal of Cardiology 8, no. 2 (1961): 178–83, https://doi.org/10.1016/0002-9149(61)90203-X.

4 Lisa J. Staton, Mukta Panda, Ian Chen, Inginia Genao, James Kurz, Mark Pasanen, et al., "When Race Matters: Disagreement in Pain Perception Between Patients and Their Physicians in Primary Care," Journal of the National Medical Association 99, no. 5 (May 2007): 532–38, https:// pmc.ncbi.nlm.nih.gov/articles/PMC2576060.

5 Ronald Wyatt, "Pain and Ethnicity," AMA Journal of Ethics 15, no. 5 (May 2013): 449–54, https://doi.org/10.1001/virtualmentor.2013.15 .5.pfor1-1305.

6 Bridgett Rahim-Williams, Joseph L. Riley, Ameenah K. Williams, and Roger B. Fillingim, "A Quantitative Review of Ethnic Group Differences

in Experimental Pain Response: Do Biology, Psychology, and Culture Matter?" Pain Medicine 13, no. 4 (April 2012): 522–40, https://doi.org /10.1111/j.1526-4637.2012.01336.x.

7 Vanessa Grubbs, "Researchers Seek Reproductive Justice for Black Women," California Health Care Foundation, September 25, 2020, www .chcf.org/blog/researchers-seek-reproductive-justice-black-women.

8 "2020 Edition—Quality of Care: Maternal Health and Childbirth," California Health Care Foundation, June 26, 2020, www.chcf.org/wp-content /uploads/2020/03/QualityCareAlmanacMaternalHealth2020.pdf

9 Dána-Ain Davis, *Reproductive Injustice: Racism, Pregnancy, and Premature Birth* (New York University Press, 2020).

10 Serena Williams, "How Serena Williams Saved Her Own Life," *Elle*, April 5, 2022, www.elle.com/life-love/a39586444/how-serena-williams-saved -her-own-life.

11 Dakin Andone, "A Black Doctor Died of Covid-19 Weeks After Accusing Hospital Staff of Racist Treatment," CNN, December 25, 2020, https://www .cnn.com/2020/12/24/us/black-doctor-susan-moore-covid-19/index.html.

12 Carolyn Crist and Lindsay Kalter, "JAMA Podcast on Racism in Medicine Faces Backlash," *Hospitalist*, March 5, 2021, https://www.the-hospitalist .org/hospitalist/article/236777/diversity-medicine/jama-podcast-racism -medicine-faces-backlash.

13 Sally Satel, PC, M.D.: *How Political Correctness is Corrupting Medicine* (Basic Books, 2000)

CHAPTER 6
DIVERSITY AND THE SOCIAL DETERMINANTS OF SUCCESS

1 Vanessa Grubbs, unpublished data from the National Study of Resident Physicians' Disciplinary Experiences, Black Doc Village, 2024.

2 N. C. Wang, "Diversity, Inclusion, and Equity: Evolution of Race and Ethnicity Considerations for the Cardiology Workforce in the United States of America from 1969 to 2019," *Journal of the American Heart*

Association 9, no. 7 (2020): e015959, https://doi.org/10.1161/jaha
.120.015959.

3 "Wang Paper Is Wrong: Diversity, Equity and Inclusiveness in Medicine
and Cardiology Are Important and Necessary," American Heart Association, August 5, 2020, https://newsroom.heart.org/news/wang-paper
-is-wrong-diversity-equity-and-inclusiveness-in-medicine-and-cardiology
-are-important-and-necessary.

4 "Retraction to: Diversity, Inclusion, and Equity: Evolution of Race and Ethnicity Considerations for the Cardiology Workforce in the United States of
America from 1969 to 2019," *Journal of the American Heart Association* 9,
no. 20 (August 2020), https://doi.org/10.1161/jaha.119.014602.

5 Association of American Medical Colleges, *Using MCAT Data in 2024
Medical Student Selection* (Washington, DC: AAMC, 2023), www.aamc
.org/media/18901/download.

6 Vanessa Grubbs, "Diversity, Equity, and Inclusion That Matter," *New
England Journal of Medicine* 383, no. 4 (July 2020), https://doi.org/10.1056
/nejmpv2022639.

7 Vanessa Grubbs, "CMS Must Act to Ensure a Diverse Physician Workforce," *Healthcare Business Today*, June 13, 2023, www.healthcarebusiness
today.com/cms-must-act-to-ensure-a-diverse-physician-workforce.

8 Elizabeth Arias, Jiaquan Xu, and Kenneth Kochanek, "United States Life
Tables, 2021," *National Vital Statistics Reports* 72, no. 12 (2023): 1–64,
www.cdc.gov/nchs/data/nvsr/nvsr72/nvsr72-12.pdf.

9 Grubbs, "Diversity, Equity, and Inclusion."

CHAPTER 7

HOW CAN MEDICINE BE RACIST

1 Institute of Medicine, *Unequal Treatment: Confronting Racial and Ethnic
Disparities in Healthcare* (National Academies Press, 2003).

2 Stanley Goldfarb, *Take Two Aspirin and Call Me by My Pronouns: Why
Turning Doctors into Social Justice Warriors Is Destroying American Medicine*
(Bombardier Books, 2022), https://doi.org/10.17226/12875.

3 Crist and Kalter, "JAMA Podcast on Racism."

4 ARIC Investigators, "The Atherosclerosis Risk in Communities (ARIC) Study: Design and Objectives," *American Journal of Epidemiology* 129, no. 4 (April 1989): 687–702, https://doi.org/10.1093/oxfordjournals.aje .a115184.

5 "Columbia University & Slavery," Columbia University & Slavery, n.d., accessed November 14, 2024, https://columbiaandslavery.columbia.edu.

6 Craig Steven Wilder, *Ebony and Ivy: Race, Slavery, and the Troubled History of America's Universities* (Bloomsbury, 2013).

7 "Slavery and Justice Report," Brown & Slavery & Justice, n.d., accessed November 14, 2024, https://slaveryandjustice.brown.edu/report.

8 Dakin Andone and Evan Simko-Bednarski, "Columbia University Will Remove Slave Owner's Name from Dormitory," *CNN*, August 31, 2020, www.cnn.com/2020/08/30/us/columbia-university-slave-owner-dorm -name-trnd/index.html.

9 Raymond Givens (Assistant Professor, Emory University School of Medicine), in discussion with the author, September 3, 2022.

10 Jocelyn Grzeszczak, "Columbia University Renames Medical School Dorm Over Its Ties to Slavery," *Newsweek*, August 29, 2020, www.newsweek .com/columbia-university-renames-medical-school-dorm-over-its-ties -slavery-1528560.

11 Washington, *Medical Apartheid*.

12 Seshat Mack (Resident Physician, Icahn School of Medicine at Mount Sinai), in discussion with the author, February 16, 2022.

13 Robert B. Baker, Harriet A. Washington, Ololade Olakanmi, Todd L. Savitt, Elizabeth A. Jacobs, Eddie Hoover, et al., "African American Physicians and Organized Medicine, 1846-1968: Origins of a Racial Divide," *JAMA* 300, no. 3 (2008): 306-13, https://doi.org/10.1001/jama.300.3.306., https://doi .org/10.1001/virtualmentor.2014.16.6.mhst1-1406.

14 Abraham Flexner, *Medical Education in the United States and Canada: A Report to the Carnegie Foundation for the Advancement of Teaching*, 1910, http://archive.carnegiefoundation.org/publications/pdfs/elibrary/Carnegie _Flexner_Report.pdf.

CHAPTER 9
LACK OF PROFESSIONALISM

1 "Race and Criminal Justice," American Civil Liberties Union, September 18, 2024, www.aclu.org/issues/racial-justice/race-and-criminal-justice.

2 "2020–21 Civil Rights Data Collection: Student Discipline and School Climate in U.S. Public Schools," Office for Civil Rights, US Department of Education, November 2023, www.ed.gov/media/document/crdc -discipline-school-climate-reportpdf.

3 "Diversity and Inclusion in Graduate Medical Education," Accreditation Council for Graduate Medical Education, 2019, https://southernhospital medicine.org/wp-content/uploads/2019/10/McDade-ACGME-SHM -Presentation-McDade-Final.pdf.

4 Usha Lee McFarling, "'It Was Stolen from Me': Black Doctors Are Forced Out of Training Programs at Far Higher Rates than White Residents," *STAT*, June 20, 2022, www.statnews.com/2022/06/20/black-doctors -forced-out-of-training-programs-at-far-higher-rates-than-white-residents.

5 "Milestones Guidebook for Residents and Fellows," Accreditation Council for Graduate Medical Education, 2020, www.acgme-i.org/globalassets /acgme-international/milestones/milestonesguidebookforresidents fellows.pdf.

6 "New AAMC Report Shows Continuing Projected Physician Shortage," Association of American Medical Colleges, March 21, 2024, www.aamc .org/news/press-releases/new-aamc-report-shows-continuing-projected -physician-shortage.

7 Grubbs, unpublished data (2024).

8 Vanessa Grubbs, "Perspective: Racism in Academic Medicine Is Hindering Progress Toward Health Equity," California Health Care Foundation, February 17, 2023, www.chcf.org/publication/perspective-racism-academic -medicine-hindering-progress-toward-health-equity.

9 *Kaiser Permanente Bernard J. Tyson School of Medicine, Inc.*, National Labor Relations Board, case number 21-CA-273372, accessed November 14, 2024, www.nlrb.gov/case/21-CA-273372.

10 Uché Blackstock, "Why Black Doctors like Me Are Leaving Faculty Positions in Academic Medical Centers," *STAT*, January 16, 2020, www.statnews .com/2020/01/16/black-doctors-leaving-faculty-positions-academic -medical-centers.

11 Uché Blackstock, *Legacy: A Black Physician Reckons with Racism in Medicine* (Viking, 2024).

CHAPTER 10
PLACEBO

1 Dictionary app, Apple Inc., s.v. "placebo," accessed November 24, 2024.

2 Grubbs, "Racism in Academic Medicine."

3 "American Hospital Association, *Diversity and Disparities: A Benchmarking Study of U.S. Hospitals in 2015* (American Hospital Association, 2016), https://web.archive.org/web/20200307072638/http://www.diversity connection.org/diversityconnection/leadershipconferences/2016%20 Conference%20Docs%20and%20Images/Diverity_Disparities2016 _final.pdf.

4 American Hospital Association, *Diversity and Disparities*.

5 "Advancing Health Equity: A Guide to Language, Narrative and Concepts," American Medical Association, n.d., accessed November 14, 2024, www.ama-assn.org/about/ama-center-health-equity/advancing-health -equity-guide-language-narrative-and-concepts-0.

6 Faculty Salary Equity at U.S. Medical Schools by Gender and Race/Ethnicity," Association of American Medical Colleges, October 2021, https:// store.aamc.org/downloadable/download/sample/sample_id/453/.

7 Donna K. Ginther, Walter T. Schaffer, Joshua Schnell, Beth Masimore, Faye Liu, Laurel L Haak, and Raynard Kington, "Race, Ethnicity, and NIH Research Awards," *Science* 333, no. 6045 (August 2011): 1015–19, https://doi.org/10.1126/science.1196783.

8 Usha Lee McFarling, "'Health Equity Tourists': How White Scholars Are Colonizing Research on Health Disparities," *STAT*, September 23, 2021,

www.statnews.com/2021/09/23/health-equity-tourists-white-scholars
-colonizing-health-disparities-research.

9 Grubbs, "Racism in Academic Medicine."

10 "CHCF Health Care Leadership Program," California Health Care Foundation, n.d., accessed October 31, 2024, www.chcf.org/program/chcf
-health-care-leadership-program.

11 Malcolm X, "Malcolm X - The most disrespected person in America is
the black woman," posted October 20, 2022, by Trey Evans, YouTube, 26
sec., www.youtube.com/watch?v=0VW9CQSOAPk.

CHAPTER 11
HUMILITY

1 Melanie Tervalon and Jann Murray-García, "Cultural Humility Versus
Cultural Competence: A Critical Distinction in Defining Physician Training Outcomes in Multicultural Education," *Journal of Health Care for the
Poor and Underserved* 9, no. 2 (May 1998): 117–25, https://doi.org/10
.1353/hpu.2010.0233.

CONCLUSION
REALITY

1 Blackpast, "(1857) Frederick Douglass, 'If There Is No Struggle, There Is
No Progress'," BlackPast.org, January 25, 2007, www.blackpast.org/african
-american-history/1857-frederick-douglass-if-there-no-struggle-there
-no-progress/.

2 Malcolm X, "Malcolm X- On Progress," posted April 21, 2008, by
mrholtshistory, YouTube, 20 sec., https://youtu.be/cReCQE8B5nY?si=
wp9sHIKwSXnLk9Ud.

3 David A. Ansari, Neera R. Jain, Constance R. Tucker, and Jennifer Karlin,
"When I Say ... Haunted Curriculum," *Medical Education*, October 16,
2024, https://doi.org/10.1111/medu.15537.

4 Usha Lee McFarling and Katie Palmer, "Inside the Bruising Battle to Purge Race from a Kidney Disease Calculator," *STAT*, September 5, 2024, www.statnews.com/2024/09/05/embedded-bias-part-3-kidney-disease -egfr-blood-test-racial-bias-kidney-transplant-list.

5 Keyerra Charles, Mary Jane Lewis, Elizabeth Montgomery, and Morgan Reid, "The 2021 Chronic Kidney Disease Epidemiology Collaboration Race-Free Estimated Glomerular Filtration Rate Equations in Kidney Disease: Leading the Way in Ending Disparities," *Health Equity* 8, no. 1 (January 2024): 39–45, https://doi.org/10.1089/heq.2023.0038.

6 Nathaniel Wesley Jr., *Black Hospitals in America: History, Contributions and Demise: A Comprehensive Review of the History, Contributions and Demise of the More Than 500 Black Hospitals of the 20th Century* (NRW Associates Publications, 2010).

7 Vanessa Grubbs, "The Gift I Didn't Realize I Needed," California Health Care Foundation, April 10, 2024, www.chcf.org/blog/gift-didnt-realize -needed.

8 Cerdeña, Grubbs, et al., "Genomic Supremacy."

INDEX

S

T

U

ABOUT THE AUTHOR

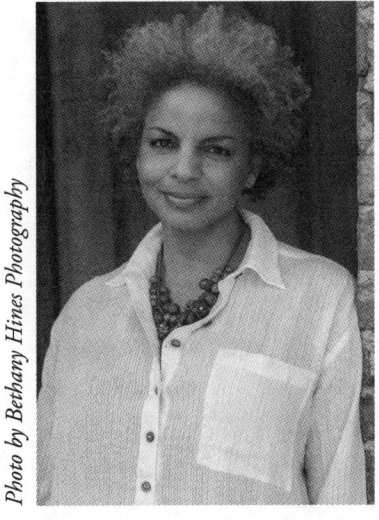

Dr. Vanessa Grubbs is an internist, nephrologist, kidney donor, physician-scientist, and author of *Hundreds of Interlaced Fingers: A Kidney Doctor's Search for the Perfect Match.* Dr. Grubbs is from Spring Lake, North Carolina. She is a Duke University undergraduate and medical school alum and completed her nephrology specialty training at UCSF, where she became a faculty member. While maintaining a clinical and research practice, she distinguished herself as a leading voice in nephrology, palliative care, and racial disparities. She left UCSF in 2019 but continues to publish in medical journals and speak at academic institutions. Currently, Dr. Grubbs is a primary care physician, runs "Real Kidney Talk with The People's Nephrologist" on YouTube, and, in 2022, founded Black Doc Village, a nonprofit organization dedicated to actively advocating for Black trainees and physicians. She lives in Oakland, California, with her husband, and 2005 recipient of her left kidney, Robert Phillips.

ABOUT NORTH ATLANTIC BOOKS

North Atlantic Books (NAB) is an independent, nonprofit publisher committed to a bold exploration of the relationships between mind, body, spirit, and nature. Founded in 1974, NAB aims to nurture a holistic view of the arts, sciences, humanities, and healing. To make a donation or to learn more about our books, authors, events, and newsletter, please visit www.northatlanticbooks.com.